KETO AIRFRYER COOKBOOK

400 HEALTHY AND FAST LOW CARBS RECIPES FOR A RAPID WEIGHT LOSS AND FAT BURN.

Patricia Burrows

Copyright © 2020 by Patricia Burrows

All right reserved. No part of this publication may be reproduced in any form without permission in writing form the publisher, except for brief quotations used for publishable articles or reviews.

Legal Disclaimer

The information contained in this book and its contents is not designed to replace any form of medical or professional advice; and is not meant to replace the need for independent medical, financial, legal, or other professional advice or service that may require. The content and information in this book have been provided for educational and entertainment purposes only.

The content and information contained in this book have been compiled from sources deemed reliable, and they are accurate to the best of the Author's knowledge, information and belief.

However, the Author cannot guarantee its accuracy and validity and therefore cannot be held liable for any errors and/or omissions.

Further, changes are periodically made to this book as needed. Where appropriate and/or necessary, you must consult a professional (including but not limited to your doctor, attorney, financial advisor, or other such professional) before using any of the suggested remedies, techniques, and/or information in this book.

Upon using this book's contents and information, you agree to hold harmless the Author from any damaged, costs and expenses, including any legal fees potentially resulting from the application of any of the information in this book. This disclaimer applies to any loss, damages, or injury caused by the use and application of this book's content, whether directly and indirectly, whether for breach of contract, tort, negligence, personal injury, criminal intent, or under any other circumstances.

You agree to accept all risks of using the information presented in this book. You agree that by continuing to read this book, where appropriate and/or necessary, you shall consult a professional (including but not limited to your doctor, attorney, financial advisor, or other such professional) before remedies, techniques, and/or information in this book.

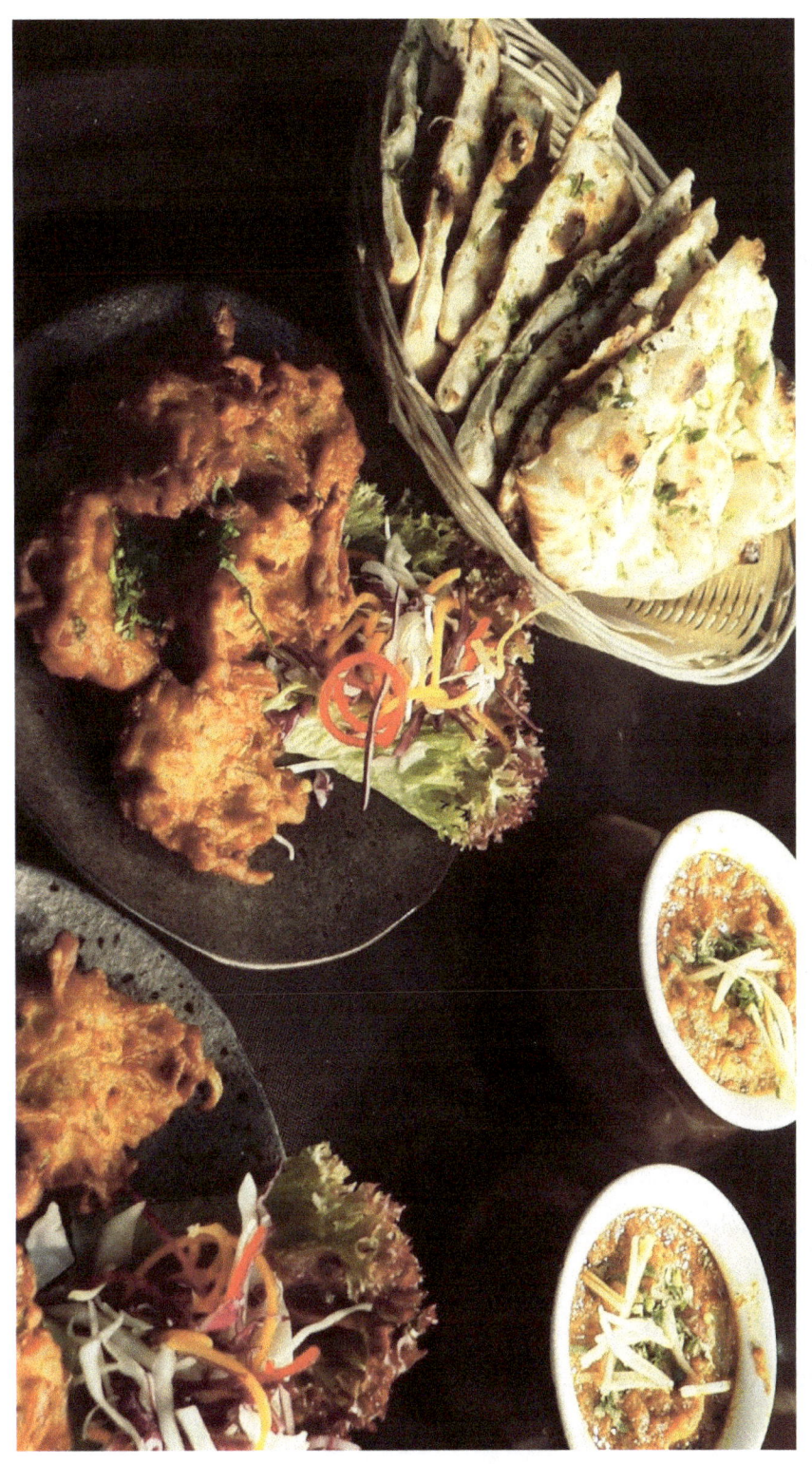

TABLE OF CONTENTS

Breakfast **18**

    Bacon-and-Eggs Avocado 18

    Eggs and Ham Avocado 19

    Baked Golden Biscuits 19

    Easy Omelet 20

    Cheesy Breakfast Sammies 21

    Patties with Tzatziki 22

    Savory Bagels 23

    Cheesy Danish 24

    Sausage Cheese Biscuit 26

    Chocolate Chip Muffin 27

    Blueberry Muffin 27

    Golden Muffin 28

    Cheesy Bacon Calzones 28

    Air Fried Ramekin 29

    Quick Omelet 30

    Tomato and Spinach Egg 31

    Sausage Egg Cup 31

    Cheesy Ham Egg 32

    Cheesy Roll 32

    Cheesy Omelet 33

    Air Fried Cheese Soufflés 34

    Bacon and Cheese Quiche 34

    Sausage Cheese Meatball 35

    Sausage Burger with Avocado 35

    Bacon Cheese Pizza 36

    Cheesy Pepperoni Egg 37

    Pecan Granola 37

    Broccoli Frittata 38

    Lemony Cake 38

Aromatic Cake 39

Cheesy Cauliflower Hash Browns 40

Cheesy Sausage Pepper 40

Cheesy Egg 41

Bacon Cheese Egg with Avocado 41

Cheesy Avocado Cauliflower 42

Air Fried Spaghetti Squash 43

Lettuce Wrap with Bacon 43

Pork Sausage Eggs With Mustard Sauce 44

Air Fried Mushroon with Tomato 45

Mushroom Frittata 46

Turkey Sausage 46

Appetizers and Snacks 48

Cauliflower with Buffalo Sauce 48

Cheesy Bacon-Wrapped Jalapeño 48

Prosciutto Cheese Asparagus Roll 49

Cheesy Mushroom 49

Three Cheese Dip 50

Cheese Chicken Dip 50

Beef and Bacon Cheese Dip 51

Cheesy Spinach Artichoke Dip 52

Cheesy Pizza Crust 52

Sausage and Bacon Cheese Pizza 53

Air Fried Almond 53

Cheesy Chicken with Bacon 54

Beef Jerky 55

Pepperoni Cheese Roll 55

Spinach Turkey Meatball 56

Cheesy Calamari Rings 57

Bacon-Wrapped Onion Rings 57

Bacon-Wrapped Cabbage Bites 58

Cheesy Chicken Wings 59

Air Fried Chicken Wings 59

Golden Pork Egg 60

- Bacon Jalapeño Cheese Bread 61
- Cheesy Bacon Pepper 61
- Prosciutto-Wrapped Guacamole Rings 62
- Cheesy Pork Rind Tortillas 63
- Cheesy Pork and Chicken 64
- Pork Cheese Sticks 64
- Cheesy Cauliflower Buns 65
- Bacon Cauliflower Skewers 66
- Crispy Cheese Salami Roll-Ups 66
- Cheesy Zucchini Fries 67
- Aromatic Avocado Fries 67
- Cheesy Pickle Spear 68
- Crispy Pepperoni Chips 69
- Vinegary Pork Belly Chips 69
- Air Fried Kale Chips 70
- Prosciutto Pierogi 71
- Air Fried Brussels Sprout 72
- Savory Eggplant 72
- Golden Cheese Crisps 73
- Broccoli Fries with Spicy Dip 73
- Cheesy Broccoli 74
- Spinach Melts with Chilled Sauce 75
- Aromatic Bacon Shrimp 76
- Roasted Zucchini 76
- Cheesy Meatball 77
- Pork Meatball 78
- Beef Cheese Burger 78
- Cheesy Chicken Nuggets 79
- Crisp Cauliflower 80
- Roast Chicken with Teriyaki Sauce 80
- Zucchini and Bacon Cheese Cake 82
- Cheesy Tomato Chips 82
- Air Fried Bell Pepper 83
- Baked Spinach Chips 84

Scallops and Bacon Kabobs 84

Bacon and Egg Bites 85

Side Dishes **87**

Kohlrabi Fries 87

Air Fried Bok Choy 87

Brussels Sprouts with Pecan 88

Brussels Sprouts with Bacon 88

Bacon-Wrapped Asparagus 89

Air Fried Asparagus 89

Cheesy Asparagus 90

Cheesy Bean Mushroon Casserole 91

Crispy Green Beans 91

Zucchini Fritters 93

Zucchini and Tomato Boats 93

Air Fried Cauliflower 94

Cheesy Cauliflower Tots 95

Cauliflower with Lime Juice 95

Cheesy Cauliflower Rice Balls 96

Cheese Cauliflower Mash 97

Broccoli with Sesame Dressing 97

Cheesy Broccoli with Bacon 98

Golden Broccoli Salad 98

Tomato Salad with Arugula 99

Sausage-Stuffed Mushroom Caps 101

Air Fried Mushroom 101

Roasted Eggplant 102

Air Fried Cabbage 102

Pork and Onion Rings 103

Cheesy Spinach Poppers 103

Roasted Salsa 104

Vegetarian Mains **105**

Zucchini Cheese Tart 106

Cauliflower with Cheese 107

Cauliflower Steak With Gremolata 107

Broccoli-Cheese Fritters 108

Air Fried Tofu 109

Cheesy Mushroom Soufflés 110

Spinach Cheese Casserole 110

Roasted Spaghetti Squash 111

Cheesy Zucchini 111

Zucchini and Mushroom Kebab 112

Eggplant with Tomato and Cheese 113

Roast Eggplant and Zucchini Bites 114

Cheesy Zucchini and Spinach 114

Cheese Stuffed Zucchini 115

Cheese Stuffed Pepper 115

Air Fried Cheesy Mushroom 116

Cheesy Celery Croquettes with Chive Mayo 117

Cauliflower Cheese Fritters 118

Broccoli with Garlic Sauce 118

Air Fried Asparagus and Broccoli 119

Poultry 120

Bacon Chicken Salad 121

Lemon Chicken 122

Savory Chicken 122

Chicken Thighs with Cilantro 123

Air Fried Chicken 124

Aromatic Chicken 124

Cheesy Chicken Breast 125

Bacon Spinach Chicken 126

Broccoli Cheese Chicken 127

Chicken Broccoli Casserole with Cheese 128

Chicken Croquettes with Creole Sauce 129

Aromatic Chicken Thigh 130

Ham Chicken with Cheese 130

Cheey Chicken with Sauce 131

Buttery Chicken 132

Air Fried Chicken 133

Spicy Cheese Chicken Roll-Up	134
Cheesy Chicken	134
Aromatic Chicken Leg	135
Chicken Legs with Turnip	136
Chicken with Brussels Sprouts	137
Roast Chicken Leg	137
Cheesy Sausage Zucchini Casserole	138
Air Fried Chicken Drumettes	139
Chicken Wing with Piri Piri Sauce	139
Creamy Chicken	140
Cheese Chicken Burgers	141
Aromatic Chicken with Cauliflower	142
White Wine Chicken Breast	143
Air Fried Cheesy Chicken	143
Chicken Vegetable with Cheese	144
Cheesy Chicken with Bacon	145
Chicken with Bacon and Tomato	145
Spicy Chicken	146
Air Fried Chicken Kebabs	147
Chicken Nuggets	149
Aromatic Chicken Thighs	150
Savory Hen	150
Quick Chicken Breast	151
Chicken Drumsticks	152
Cheesy Turkey Meatball	153
Air Fried Turkey Breast	154
Turkey with Mustard Sauce	154
Turkey Breasts with Mustard	155
Air Fried Turkey	156
Roast Turkey	156
Turkey with Gravy	157
Air Fried Turkey and Chicken	157
Easy Turkey Drumsticks	158
Cheesy Turkey Kabobs	159

Bacon-Wrapped Turkey with Cheese 159

Turkey with Tabasco Sauce 160

Turkey Sausage with Cauliflower 161

Beef, Pork, and Lamb 162

Air Fried Flank Steak 162

Cheesy Flank Steak 162

Cheese Steak with Lettuce 163

Zucchini Noodle with Beef Meatball 164

Ribs with Chimichurri Sauce 165

Spinach Cheese Steak 166

Buttery Strip Steak 167

Steak with Butter 168

Steak with Bell Pepper 168

Cheesy Beef Burger with Mushroom 169

Roast Beef 170

Beef Steak Shallots 171

Steak with Horseradish Cream 171

Aromatic Ribeye Steak 172

Air Fried Top Chuck 173

Beef Burger 173

Roast Beef 174

Roast Beef Steaks 175

Air Fried Beef Steak 175

Beef Parboiled Sausage 176

Red Wine Rib 177

Chuck Kebab with Arugula 177

Cheesy Filet Mignon 178

Air Fried London Broil 179

Creamy Beef Steak 179

Beef Chuck with Brussels Sprouts 180

Creamy Beef Flank Steak 181

Air Fried Skirt Steak 182

Beef Sausage with Tomato Bowl 182

Loin Steak with Mayo 184

Cheesy Sirloin Steak 184
Lemony Beef Steak 185
Mushroom Sausage Biscuit 186
Cheesy Sausage Balls 187
Italian Sausage Link 188
Cheese Pork Chop 188
Bacon-Wrapped Cheese Pork 189
Pork with Lime Sauce 190
Air Fried Pork Belly 191
Roast Pork Belly 192
Air Fried Pork Meatballs 192
Onion Pork Kebabs 193
Pork Kebab with Yogurt Sauce 194
Cheesy Pork Beef Casserole 195
Savory Porterhouse Steak 195
Cheese Wine Pork Cutlets 196
Cheesy Pork Tenderloin 197
Cheese Pork Meatballs 198
Air Fried Pork Chop 198
Roast Pork Tenderloin 199
Aromatic Pork Loin Roast 199
Savory Pork Loin 200
Greens with Shallot and Bacon 201
Cheesy Pork Sausage Meatball 201
Pork Cheese Casserole 202
Baked Sauerkraut with Sausage 203
Greek Pork with Tzatziki Sauce 204
Tangy Lamb Chop 205

Fish and Seafood 206

Swordfish Skewers with Cherry Tomato 206
Air Fried Cod Fillet 207
Cod with Avocado 208
Air Fried Cod Fillets 209
Cod with Jalapeno 209

- Air Fried Cod Fillet ... 210
- Cod with Tomatillos ... 210
- White Fish with Cauliflower ... 211
- Cheesy Hake Fillet ... 211
- Cheesy Tuna ... 212
- Grilled Tuna Cake ... 213
- Tuna Steak ... 214
- Creamy Tuna Pork Casserole ... 214
- Tuna Avocado Bites ... 215
- Rockfish with Avocado Cream ... 215
- Whitefish Fillet with Green Bean ... 216
- Baked Monkfish ... 217
- Cheesy Flounder Cutlets ... 218
- Roast Swordfish Steak ... 219
- Snapper with Shallot and Tomato ... 219
- Air Fried Salmon ... 221
- Savory Salmon Fillet ... 222
- Salmon with Provolone Cheese ... 222
- Salmon with Endives ... 223
- Salmon Fritters with Zucchini ... 223
- Air Fried Salmon Fillet ... 224
- Tasty Salmon ... 224
- Salmon with Cauliflower ... 225
- Lemony Salmon ... 225
- Crispy Salmon Patties ... 226
- Air Fried Salmon ... 226
- Air Fried Catfish ... 227
- Tilapia with Pecan ... 227
- Easy Tilapia Fillet ... 228
- Savory Tilapia ... 228
- Sweet Tilapia Fillets ... 229
- Air Fried Tilapia ... 229
- Quick Tilapia ... 230
- Creamy Haddock ... 230

Mackerel with Spinach 231
Air Fried Mackerel Fillet 231
Creamy Mackerel 232
Easy Sardines 232
Bacon Halibut Steak 233
Shrimp with Romaine 233
Air Fried Shrimp 234
Savory Shrimp 235
Buttery Scallops 235
Crab Cake 236
Easy Shrimp 237
Air Fried Shrimp 238
Golden Shrimp 238
Cheesy Shrimp 239
Shrimp with Swiss Chard 240
Cheesy Crab Patties 240
Air Fried Crab Bun 241
Quick Shrimp Skewers 241
Air Fried Mussels 242
Savory Lobster Tail 242
Delicious Scallops 243
Calamari with Hot Sauce 243

Desserts 245

Chocolate Butter Cake 245
Buttery Chocolate Cake 245
Chocolate Butter Cake 246
Butter Chocolate Cake with Pecan 248
Baked Cheesecake 248
Crusted Mini Cheesecake 249
Creamy Cheese Cake 250
Air Fried Chocolate Brownies 251
Butter Cake with Cranberries 252
Buttery Monk Fruit Cookie 253
Buttery Cookie with Hazelnut 254

Hazelnut Butter Cookie 255

Walnut Butter Cookie 255

Buttery Almond Fruit Cookie 256

Butter and Chocolate Chip Cookie 257

Blueberry Cream Flan 257

Air Fried Muffin 258

Homemade Muffin 259

Creamy Pecan Bar 259

Lime Bar 260

Macadamia Bar 261

Zucchini Bread 261

Creamy Vanilla Scones 262

Homemade Mint Pie 262

Cheese Keto Balls 263

Pecan Butter Cookie 264

Golden Doughnut Holes 264

Chocolate Chips Soufflés 265

Creamy Strawberry Pecan Pie 266

Chocolate Chip Cookie Cake 266

Prep time: 5 minutes | Cook time: 15 minutes | Serves 8 266

Homemade Pretzels 267

Pecan Chocolate Brownies 267

Butter Cheesecake 268

Golden Cheese Cookie 269

Toasted Coconut Flakes 270

Cheesy Cream Cake 270

Cheese Monkey Bread 271

Cheesy Cream Puffs 272

Introduction

There are many diets out there that promise to help you lose weight. Some of them even work! However, this doesn't explain the large number of dieters who fail to hit their goals. Why is this? Is dieting really that hard? Or is there something else going on that causes them to miss their goals?

The fact is that dieting is hard. When you're trying to get healthy and lose weight, you're trying to undo years' worth of habits that won't suddenly disappear. This is why many dieters report gaining the weight they once lost right back. The experience of dieting stresses them to such an extent that once they stop dieting, they start binge eating and undo all the good work they've done.

There is no single right way to diet. The key to dieting success is to follow a good method and to then make it as easy as possible to follow what needs to be done. The thing to keep in mind is that not all diets are easy to follow. This isn't because of some complexity in them. It's just that some people are used to eating in the way the diet recommends.

The ketogenic diet is one such example. The diet calls for a very small number of carbs to be eaten. This means food such as rice, pasta, and other starchy vegetables like potatoes are off the menu. Even relaxed versions of the keto diet minimize carbs to a large extent and this compromises the goals of many dieters. They end up having to exert large amounts of willpower to follow the diet.

This doesn't do them any favors since willpower is like a muscle. At some point, it tires and this is when the dieter goes right back to their old pattern of eating. I have personal experience with this. In terms of health benefits, the keto diet offers the most. The reduction of carbs forces your body to mobilize fat and this results in automatic fat loss and better health.

While the benefits were massive, I couldn't stick to the diet for long periods of time due to lifestyle difficulties. The fact is that when I started out on the keto diet, I was extremely busy and didn't have time to spend in the kitchen. Not only did I lack the time, I didn't have any inclination to be in there as well. As far as I was concerned, the best recipe was one that could create a great dish in a few minutes!

If you've followed the keto diet you probably know how most recipes work. Most of them involve grilling and baking. The protein is then put into a salad and that's your meal. While the novelty factor managed to keep me excited for meals, this soon wore off. There's only so much salad a person can eat before they become disgusting! No amount of fancy vegetables and meat could make them more attractive.

I needed a better solution.

Enter the Air Fryer

When I first stumbled into the air fryer I had serious second thoughts. After all, in order to fry something you need to coat it with tons of grease and bread crumbs. You then have to dip it into even more oil to fry it. How could frying possibly help me get healthy and keep me on track to hit my weight loss goals?

I was in a particularly dire moment at that time. I was about to switch off the keto diet once again because I simply could not manage to prep my meals and cook them ahead of time. I needed a quick and simple solution that wouldn't compromise my health goals. I figured I had nothing to lose so why not give it a shot.

The air fryer's technology might make it sound like a really complicated piece of engineering. It's pretty simple once you understand it. All the air fryer does is pass really hot air over food. This means you don't need to coat it with excess grease or fat. In fact, you can fry food without having to coat it with oil at all.

You can enjoy traditionally fried food such as chicken tenders and nuggets with just a little bit of oil thrown into the mix. This makes it an extremely healthy option for those who are looking to hit their weight loss goals. By ingesting less harmful fat you'll manage to stay within your calorie goals. The best thing of all?

Your food cooks in literally a few minutes! This was what struck me when I first began using my air fryer. It made a few weird noises sure, but my food was ready in a minute and best of all, it was so much tastier than anything I had cooked before! You could say I've been on the air fryer bandwagon ever since!

The air fryer isn't a complete solution to all of your diet-related issues. However, it makes it extremely simple for you to follow the keto diet. Think about it. If you don't need to plan ahead or constantly think about what you need to eat all the time, you're more likely to fall into a healthy pattern of eating.

Following the keto diet will become automatic for you, much like brushing your teeth is. You don't think about how you need to do this do you? So why not adopt the same principle when trying to diet? Make it as simple as possible for you to execute and you'll never have to worry about eating the wrong thing or eating something you're unhappy with.

The keto diet has innumerable health benefits for you. However, you need to set things up in such a way so that you give yourself no way to violate its guidelines. The air fryer helps you do this easily and all of the recipes in here are proof of that. There are 500 recipes in here so there's more than enough for you to choose from.

Take your time choosing the ones that appeal to you the most. I'm positive you'll find sticking to your diet so much easier once you've adopted the air fryer lifestyle!

The Diet as a Lifestyle

I'll confess that I made a few mistakes when I first adopted the diet. My partner and I found it difficult to adjust to the new way of cooking. We were so used to eating carb heavy meals that at first, eating a salad didn't seem enough. "There's no way that'll fill me up!" I thought.

While the going was tough initially, things became a lot easier as time went on. I'm not saying you need to survive on just salads. It's just that every diet is difficult to adopt at first. You're not just fighting against your taste buds. You're trying to change eating habits that have been ingrained in you for a long time. These habits aren't easily overturned.

These days we find it really simple to cook our food and we spend very little time prepping it. As a result, our health has improved and we're much happier. How did we manage to overcome our hurdles? The secret to all of this has been our air fryer. At first, prepping food took too much time and truth be told, neither of us are keen cooks.

We wanted to eat food that was tasty and easily prepared. However, this is tough to do if you aren't someone who's a passionate chef. The air fryer rescued us since it offered a simple and easy way for us to cook our food and to cook it in a healthy way. Now, the word "fryer" doesn't associate itself with health. It probably conjures images of greasy food that's extremely unhealthy in your mind.

This is not what the air fryer does. If anything, it's the opposite. The air fryer uses extremely hot air to fry food and it doesn't need oil to work. You can coat your food with a light layer of grease but you don't need anywhere near the tubs of hot oil that traditional frying methods need.

All of the recipes in this book come from our experience as amateur cooks with an air fryer. We really wanted to create recipes that can be cooked in small quantities and can be shared by two people. Existing cookbooks seem to contain recipes that are meant to be prepared in large batches. This is not the case here.

All of these 600 recipes can be whipped up in no time and best of all, they're Mediterranean-diet friendly and delicious! No more worrying about what to cook tomorrow or how you're going to prep something! All you need to do is buy ingredients in the portions described in here and you'll have a delicious meal ready for two.

Feel free to mix and match the recipes you see in here and play around with them. Eating is supposed to be fun! Unfortunately, we've associated fun eating with unhealthy food. This doesn't have to be the case. The air fryer, combined with the Mediterranean diet, will make your mealtimes fun-filled again and full of taste. There's no grease and messy cleanups to deal with anymore.

Are you excited yet? You should be! You're about to embark on a journey full of air fried goodness!

Breakfast

Bacon-and-Eggs Avocado

Prep time: 5 minutes | Cook time: 17 minutes | Serves: 1

1 large egg

1 avocado, halved, peeled, and pitted

2 slices bacon

Fresh parsley, for serving (optional)

Sea salt flakes, for garnish (optional)

1. Spray the air fryer basket with avocado oil. Preheat the air fryer to 320°F (160°C). Fill a small bowl with cool water.
2. Soft-boil the egg: Place the egg in the air fryer basket. Cook for 6 minutes for a soft yolk or 7 minutes for a cooked yolk. Transfer the egg to the bowl of cool water and let sit for 2 minutes. Peel and set aside.
3. Use a spoon to carve out extra space in the center of the avocado halves until the cavities are big enough to fit the soft-boiled egg. Place the soft-boiled egg in the center of one half of the avocado and replace the other half of the avocado on top, so the avocado appears whole on the outside.
4. Starting at one end of the avocado, wrap the bacon around the avocado to completely cover it. Use toothpicks to hold the bacon in place.
5. Place the bacon-wrapped avocado in the air fryer basket and cook for 5 minutes. Flip the avocado over and cook for another 5 minutes, or until the bacon is cooked to your liking. Serve on a bed of fresh parsley, if desired, and sprinkle with salt flakes, if desired.
6. Best served fresh. Store extras in an airtight container in the fridge for up to 4 days. Reheat in a preheated 320°F (160°C) air fryer for 4 minutes, or until heated through.

Per Serving

calories: 535 | fat: 46g | protein: 18g | carbs: 18g | net carbs: 4g | fiber: 14g

Eggs and Ham Avocado

Prep time: 5 minutes | Cook time: 10 minutes | Serves 2

1 large Hass avocado, halved and pitted

2 thin slices ham

2 large eggs

2 tablespoons chopped green onions, plus more for garnish

½ teaspoon fine sea salt

¼ teaspoon ground black pepper

¼ cup shredded Cheddar cheese (omit for dairy-free)

1. Preheat the air fryer to 400°F (205ºC).
2. Place a slice of ham into the cavity of each avocado half. Crack an egg on top of the ham, then sprinkle on the green onions, salt, and pepper.
3. Place the avocado halves in the air fryer cut side up and cook for 10 minutes, or until the egg is cooked to your desired doneness. Top with the cheese (if using) and cook for 30 seconds more, or until the cheese is melted. Garnish with chopped green onions.
4. Best served fresh. Store extras in an airtight container in the fridge for up to 4 days. Reheat in a preheated 350°F (180ºC) air fryer for a few minutes, until warmed through.

Per Serving

calories: 307 | fat: 24g | protein: 14g | carbs: 10g | net carbs: 3g | fiber: 7g

Baked Golden Biscuits

Prep time: 15 minutes | Cook time: 13 minutes | Serves 8

2 cups blanched almond flour

½ cup Swerve confectioners'-style sweetener or equivalent amount of liquid or powdered sweetener

1 teaspoon baking powder

½ teaspoon fine sea salt

¼ cup plus 2 tablespoons (¾ stick) very cold unsalted butter

¼ cup unsweetened, unflavored almond milk

1 large egg

1 teaspoon vanilla extract

3 teaspoons ground cinnamon

Glaze:

½ cup Swerve confectioners'-style sweetener or equivalent amount of powdered sweetener

¼ cup heavy cream or unsweetened, unflavored almond milk

1. Preheat the air fryer to 350°F (180ºC). Line a pie pan that fits into your air fryer with parchment paper.
2. In a medium-sized bowl, mix together the almond flour, sweetener (if powdered; do not add liquid sweetener), baking powder, and salt. Cut the butter into ½-inch squares, then use a hand mixer to work the butter into the dry ingredients. When you are done, the mixture should still have chunks of butter.
3. In a small bowl, whisk together the almond milk, egg, and vanilla extract (if using liquid sweetener, add it as well) until blended. Using a fork, stir the wet ingredients into the dry ingredients until large clumps form. Add the cinnamon and use your hands to swirl it into the dough.
4. Form the dough into sixteen 1-inch balls and place them on the prepared pan, spacing them about ½-inch apart. (If you're using a smaller air fryer, work in batches if necessary.) Bake in the air fryer until golden, 10 to 13 minutes. Remove from the air fryer and let cool on the pan for at least 5 minutes.
5. While the biscuits bake, make the glaze: Place the powdered sweetener in a small bowl and slowly stir in the heavy cream with a fork.
6. When the biscuits have cooled somewhat, dip the tops into the glaze, allow it to dry a bit, and then dip again for a thick glaze.
7. Serve warm or at room temperature. Store unglazed biscuits in an airtight container in the refrigerator for up to 3 days or in the freezer for up to a month. Reheat in a preheated 350°F (180ºC) air fryer for 5 minutes, or until warmed through, and dip in the glaze as instructed above.

Per Serving

calories: 546 | fat: 51g | protein: 14g | carbs: 13g | net carbs: 7g | fiber: 6g

Easy Omelet

Prep time: 5 minutes | Cook time: 8 minutes | Serves 1

2 large eggs

¼ cup unsweetened, unflavored almond milk

¼ teaspoon fine sea salt

⅛ teaspoon ground black pepper

¼ cup diced ham (omit for vegetarian)

¼ cup diced green and red bell peppers

2 tablespoons diced green onions, plus more for garnish

¼ cup shredded Cheddar cheese (about 1 ounce / 28g) (omit for dairy-free)

Quartered cherry tomatoes, for serving (optional)

1. Preheat the air fryer to 350°F (180ºC). Grease a 6 by 3-inch cake pan and set aside.
2. In a small bowl, use a fork to whisk together the eggs, almond milk, salt, and pepper. Add the ham, bell peppers, and green onions. Pour the mixture into the greased pan. Add the cheese on top (if using).
3. Place the pan in the basket of the air fryer. Cook for 8 minutes, or until the eggs are cooked to your liking.
4. Loosen the omelet from the sides of the pan with a spatula and place it on a serving plate. Garnish with green onions and serve with cherry tomatoes, if desired. Best served fresh.

Per Serving

calories: 476 | fat: 32g | protein: 41g | carbs: 3g | net carbs: 2g | fiber: 1g

Cheesy Breakfast Sammies

Prep time: 15 minutes | Cook time: 20 minutes | Serves 5

Biscuits:

6 large egg whites

2 cups blanched almond flour, plus more if needed

1½ teaspoons baking powder

½ teaspoon fine sea salt

¼ cup (½ stick) very cold unsalted butter (or lard for dairy-free), cut into ¼-inch pieces

Eggs:

5 large eggs

½ teaspoon fine sea salt

¼ teaspoon ground black pepper

5 (1-ounce / 28-g) slices Cheddar cheese (omit for dairy-free)

10 thin slices ham, or 4 cooked Gyro Breakfast Patties

1. Spray the air fryer basket with avocado oil. Preheat the air fryer to 350°F (180ºC). Grease two 6-inch pie pans or two baking pans that will fit inside your air fryer.
2. Make the biscuits: In a medium-sized bowl, whip the egg whites with a hand mixer until very stiff. Set aside.

3. In a separate medium-sized bowl, stir together the almond flour, baking powder, and salt until well combined. Cut in the butter. Gently fold the flour mixture into the egg whites with a rubber spatula. If the dough is too wet to form into mounds, add a few tablespoons of almond flour until the dough holds together well.

4. Using a large spoon, divide the dough into 5 equal portions and drop them about 1-inch apart on one of the greased pie pans. (If you're using a smaller air fryer, work in batches if necessary.) Place the pan in the air fryer and cook for 11 to 14 minutes, until the biscuits are golden brown. Remove from the air fryer and set aside to cool.

5. Make the eggs: Set the air fryer to 375°F (190ºC). Crack the eggs into the remaining greased pie pan and sprinkle with the salt and pepper. Place the eggs in the air fryer to cook for 5 minutes, or until they are cooked to your liking.

6. Open the air fryer and top each egg yolk with a slice of cheese (if using). Cook for another minute, or until the cheese is melted.

7. Once the biscuits are cool, slice them in half lengthwise. Place 1 cooked egg topped with cheese and 2 slices of ham in each biscuit.

8. Store leftover biscuits, eggs, and ham in separate airtight containers in the fridge for up to 3 days. Reheat the biscuits and eggs on a baking sheet in a preheated 350°F (180ºC) air fryer for 5 minutes, or until warmed through.

Per Serving

calories: 585 | fat: 46g | protein: 36g | carbs: 11g | net carbs: 6g | fiber: 5g

Patties with Tzatziki

Prep time: 10 minutes | Cook time: 20 minutes | Serves 16

Patties:

2 pounds (907 g) ground lamb or beef

½ cup diced red onions

¼ cup sliced black olives

2 tablespoons tomato purée

1 teaspoon dried oregano leaves

1 teaspoon Greek seasoning

2 cloves garlic, minced

1 teaspoon fine sea salt

Tzatziki:

1 cup full-fat sour cream

1 small cucumber, chopped

½ teaspoon fine sea salt

½ teaspoon garlic powder, or 1 clove garlic, minced

¼ teaspoon dried dill weed, or 1 teaspoon finely chopped fresh dill

FOR GARNISH/SERVING:

½ cup crumbled feta cheese (about 2 ounces)

Diced red onions

Sliced black olives

Sliced cucumbers

1. Preheat the air fryer to 350°F (180°C).
2. Place the ground lamb, onions, olives, tomato purée, oregano, Greek seasoning, garlic, and salt in a large bowl. Mix well to combine the ingredients.
3. Using your hands, form the mixture into sixteen 3-inch patties. Place about 5 of the patties in the air fryer and fry for 20 minutes, flipping halfway through. Remove the patties and place them on a serving platter. Repeat with the remaining patties.
4. While the patties cook, make the tzatziki: Place all the ingredients in a small bowl and stir well. Cover and store in the fridge until ready to serve. Garnish with ground black pepper before serving.
5. Serve the patties with a dollop of tzatziki, a sprinkle of crumbled feta cheese, diced red onions, sliced black olives, and sliced cucumbers.
6. Store leftovers in an airtight container in the refrigerator for up to 5 days or in the freezer for up to a month. Reheat the patties in a preheated 390°F (199°C) air fryer for a few minutes, until warmed through.

Per Serving

calories: 396 | fat: 31g | protein: 23g | carbs: 4g | net carbs: 3g | fiber: 1g

Savory Bagels

Prep time: 15 minutes | Cook time: 14 minutes | Serves 6

1¾ cups shredded Mozzarella cheese or goat cheese

2 tablespoons unsalted butter or coconut oil

1 large egg, beaten

1 tablespoon apple cider vinegar

1 cup blanched almond flour

1 tablespoon baking powder

⅛ teaspoon fine sea salt

1½ teaspoons everything bagel seasoning

1. Make the dough: Put the Mozzarella and butter in a large microwave-safe bowl and microwave for 1 to 2 minutes, until the cheese is entirely melted. Stir well. Add the egg and vinegar. Using a hand mixer on medium, combine well. Add the almond flour, baking powder, and salt and, using the mixer, combine well.
2. Lay a piece of parchment paper on the countertop and place the dough on it. Knead it for about 3 minutes. The dough should be a little sticky but pliable. (If the dough is too sticky, chill it in the refrigerator for an hour or overnight.)
3. Preheat the air fryer to 350°F (180ºC). Spray a baking sheet or pie pan that will fit into your air fryer with avocado oil.
4. Divide the dough into 6 equal portions. Roll 1 portion into a log that is 6-inches long and about ½-inch thick. Form the log into a circle and seal the edges together, making a bagel shape. Repeat with the remaining portions of dough, making 6 bagels.
5. Place the bagels on the greased baking sheet. Spray the bagels with avocado oil and top with everything bagel seasoning, pressing the seasoning into the dough with your hands.
6. Place the bagels in the air fryer and cook for 14 minutes, or until cooked through and golden brown, flipping after 6 minutes.
7. Remove the bagels from the air fryer and allow them to cool slightly before slicing them in half and serving. Store leftovers in an airtight container in the fridge for up to 4 days or in the freezer for up to a month.

Per Serving

calories: 224 | fat: 19g | protein: 12g | carbs: 4g | net carbs: 2g | fiber: 2g

Cheesy Danish

Prep time: 15 minutes | Cook time: 20 minutes | Serves 6

Pastry:

3 large eggs

¼ teaspoon cream of tartar

¼ cup vanilla-flavored egg white protein powder

¼ cup Swerve confectioners'-style sweetener or equivalent amount of liquid or powdered sweetener (see here), or 1 teaspoon stevia glycerite

3 tablespoons full-fat sour cream (or coconut cream for dairy-free)

1 teaspoon vanilla extract

Filling:

4 ounces (113 g) cream cheese (½ cup) (or Kite Hill brand cream cheese style spread for dairy-free), softened

2 large egg yolks (from above)

¼ cup Swerve confectioners'-style sweetener or equivalent amount of liquid or powdered sweetener, or ½ teaspoon stevia glycerite

1 teaspoon vanilla extract

¼ teaspoon ground cinnamon

Drizzle:

1 ounce (28 g) cream cheese (2 tablespoons) (or Kite Hill brand cream cheese style spread for dairy-free), softened

1 tablespoon Swerve confectioners'-style sweetener or equivalent amount of liquid or powdered sweetener, or 1 drop stevia glycerite

1 tablespoon unsweetened, unflavored almond milk (or heavy cream for nut-free)

1. Preheat the air fryer to 300°F (150ºC). Spray a casserole dish that will fit in your air fryer with avocado oil.
2. Make the pastry: Separate the eggs, putting all the whites in a large bowl, one yolk in a medium-sized bowl, and two yolks in a small bowl. Beat all the egg yolks and set aside.
3. Add the cream of tartar to the egg whites. Whip the whites with a hand mixer until very stiff, then turn the hand mixer's setting to low and slowly add the protein powder while mixing. Mix until only just combined; if you mix too long, the whites will fall. Set aside.
4. To the egg yolk in the medium-sized bowl, add the sweetener, sour cream, and vanilla extract. Mix well. Slowly pour the yolk mixture into the egg whites and gently combine. Dollop 6 equal-sized mounds of batter into the casserole dish. Use the back of a large spoon to make an indentation on the top of each mound. Set aside.
5. Make the filling: Place the cream cheese in a small bowl and stir to break it up. Add the 2 remaining egg yolks, the sweetener, vanilla extract, and cinnamon and stir until well combined. Divide the filling among the mounds of batter, pouring it into the indentations on the tops.
6. Place the Danish in the air fryer and bake for about 20 minutes, or until golden brown.
7. While the Danish bake, make the drizzle: In a small bowl, stir the cream cheese to break it up. Stir in the sweetener and almond milk. Place the mixture in a piping bag or a small resealable plastic bag with one corner snipped off. After the Danish have cooled, pipe the drizzle over the Danish.
8. Store leftovers in airtight container in the fridge for up to 4 days.

Per Serving

calories: 160 | fat: 12g | protein: 8g | carbs: 2g | net carbs: 1g | fiber: 1g

Sausage Cheese Biscuit

Prep time: 20 minutes | Cook time: 30 minutes | Serves 4

Filling:

10 ounces (283 g) bulk pork sausage, crumbled

¼ cup minced onions

2 cloves garlic, minced

½ teaspoon fine sea salt

½ teaspoon ground black pepper

1 (8-ounce / 227-g) package cream cheese (or Kite Hill brand cream cheese style spread for dairy-free), softened

¾ cup beef or chicken broth

Biscuits:

3 large egg whites

¾ cup blanched almond flour

1 teaspoon baking powder

¼ teaspoon fine sea salt

2½ tablespoons very cold unsalted butter, cut into ¼-inch pieces

Fresh thyme leaves, for garnish

1. Preheat the air fryer to 400°F (205ºC).
2. Place the sausage, onions, and garlic in a 7-inch pie pan. Using your hands, break up the sausage into small pieces and spread it evenly throughout the pie pan. Season with the salt and pepper. Place the pan in the air fryer and cook for 5 minutes.
3. While the sausage cooks, place the cream cheese and broth in a food processor or blender and purée until smooth.
4. Remove the pork from the air fryer and use a fork or metal spatula to crumble it more. Pour the cream cheese mixture into the sausage and stir to combine. Set aside.
5. Make the biscuits: Place the egg whites in a medium-sized mixing bowl or the bowl of a stand mixer and whip with a hand mixer or stand mixer until stiff peaks form.
6. In a separate medium-sized bowl, whisk together the almond flour, baking powder, and salt, then cut in the butter. When you are done, the mixture should still have chunks of butter. Gently fold the flour mixture into the egg whites with a rubber spatula.
7. Use a large spoon or ice cream scoop to scoop the dough into 4 equal-sized biscuits, making sure the butter is evenly distributed. Place the biscuits on top of the sausage and cook in the air fryer for 5 minutes, then turn the heat down to 325°F (163ºC) and cook for

another 17 to 20 minutes, until the biscuits are golden brown. Serve garnished with fresh thyme leaves.

8. Store leftovers in an airtight container in the refrigerator for up to 3 days. Reheat in a preheated 350°F (180°C) air fryer for 5 minutes, or until warmed through.

Per Serving

calories: 623 | fat: 55g | protein: 23g | carbs: 8g | net carbs: 5g | fiber: 3g

Chocolate Chip Muffin

Prep time: 5 minutes | Cook time: 15 minutes | Makes 6 Muffins

1½ cups blanched finely ground almond flour

$1/3$ cup granular brown erythritol

4 tablespoons salted butter, melted

2 large eggs, whisked

1 tablespoon baking powder

½ cup low-carb chocolate chips

1. In a large bowl, combine all ingredients. Evenly pour batter into six silicone muffin cups greased with cooking spray.
2. Place muffin cups into air fryer basket. Adjust the temperature to 320°F (160°C) and set the timer for 15 minutes. Muffins will be golden brown when done.
3. Let muffins cool in cups 15 minutes to avoid crumbling. Serve warm.

Per Serving

calories: 329 | fat: 29g | protein: 10g | carbs: 28g | net carbs: 20g | fiber: 8g

Blueberry Muffin

Prep time: 5 minutes | Cook time: 15 minutes | Makes 6 Muffins

1½ cups blanched finely ground almond flour

½ cup granular erythritol

4 tablespoons salted butter, melted

2 large eggs, whisked

2 teaspoons baking powder

⅓ cup fresh blueberries, chopped

1. In a large bowl, combine all ingredients. Evenly pour batter into six silicone muffin cups greased with cooking spray.
2. Place muffin cups into air fryer basket. Adjust the temperature to 320°F (160°C) and set the timer for 15 minutes. Muffins should be golden brown when done.
3. Let muffins cool in cups 15 minutes to avoid crumbling. Serve warm.

Per Serving

calories:269 | fat: 24g | protein: 8g | carbs: 23g | net carbs: 20g | fiber: 3g

Golden Muffin

Prep time: 5 minutes | Cook time: 15 minutes | Makes 6 Muffins

1 cup blanched finely ground almond flour

¼ cup granular erythritol

2 tablespoons salted butter, melted

1 large egg, whisked

2 teaspoons baking powder

1 teaspoon ground allspice

1. In a large bowl, combine all ingredients. Evenly pour batter into six silicone muffin cups greased with cooking spray.
2. Place muffin cups into air fryer basket. Adjust the temperature to 320°F (160°C) and set the timer for 15 minutes. Cooked muffins should be golden brown.
3. Let muffins cool in cups 15 minutes to avoid crumbling. Serve warm.

Per Serving

calories: 160 | fat: 14g | protein: 5g | carbs: 20g | net carbs: 18g | fiber: 2g

Cheesy Bacon Calzones

Prep time: 15 minutes | Cook time: 12 minutes | Serves 4

2 large eggs

1 cup blanched finely ground almond flour

2 cups shredded Mozzarella cheese

2 ounces (57 g) cream cheese, softened and broken into small pieces

4 slices cooked sugar-free bacon, crumbled

1. Beat eggs in a small bowl. Pour into a medium nonstick skillet over medium heat and scramble. Set aside.
2. In a large microwave-safe bowl, mix flour and Mozzarella. Add cream cheese to bowl.
3. Place bowl in microwave and cook 45 seconds on high to melt cheese, then stir with a fork until a soft dough ball forms.
4. Cut a piece of parchment to fit air fryer basket. Separate dough into two sections and press each out into an 8-inch round.
5. On half of each dough round, place half of the scrambled eggs and crumbled bacon. Fold the other side of the dough over and press to seal the edges.
6. Place calzones on ungreased parchment and into air fryer basket. Adjust the temperature to 350°F (180°C) and set the timer for 12 minutes, turning calzones halfway through cooking. Crust will be golden and firm when done.
7. Let calzones cool on a cooking rack 5 minutes before serving.

Per Serving

calories: 477 | fat: 35g | protein: 28g | carbs: 10g | net carbs: 7g | fiber: 3g

Air Fried Ramekin

Prep time: 5 minutes | Cook time: 8 minutes | Serves 2

2 teaspoons unsalted butter (or coconut oil for dairy-free), for greasing the ramekins

4 large eggs

2 teaspoons chopped fresh thyme

½ teaspoon fine sea salt

¼ teaspoon ground black pepper

2 tablespoons heavy cream (or unsweetened, unflavored almond milk for dairy-free)

3 tablespoons finely grated Parmesan cheese (or Kite Hill brand chive cream cheese style spread, softened, for dairy-free)

Fresh thyme leaves, for garnish (optional)

1. Preheat the air fryer to 400°F (205ºC). Grease two 4-ounce (113-g) ramekins with the butter.
2. Crack 2 eggs into each ramekin and divide the thyme, salt, and pepper between the ramekins. Pour 1 tablespoon of the heavy cream into each ramekin. Sprinkle each ramekin with 1½ tablespoons of the Parmesan cheese.
3. Place the ramekins in the air fryer and cook for 8 minutes for soft-cooked yolks (longer if you desire a harder yolk).
4. Garnish with a sprinkle of ground black pepper and thyme leaves, if desired. Best served fresh.

Per Serving

calories: 331 | fat: 29g | protein: 16g | carbs: 2g | net carbs: 1g | fiber: 1g

Quick Omelet

Prep time: 5 minutes | Cook time: 15 minutes | Serves 2

3 large eggs

1 tablespoon salted butter, melted

¼ cup seeded and chopped green bell pepper

2 tablespoons peeled and chopped yellow onion

¼ cup chopped cooked no-sugar-added ham

¼ teaspoon salt

¼ teaspoon ground black pepper

1. Crack eggs into an ungreased 6-inch round nonstick baking dish. Mix in butter, bell pepper, onion, ham, salt, and black pepper.
2. Place dish into air fryer basket. Adjust the temperature to 320°F (160ºC) and set the timer for 15 minutes. The eggs will be fully cooked and firm in the middle when done.
3. Slice in half and serve warm on two medium plates.

Per Serving

calories: 201 | fat: 14g | protein: 13g | carbs: 3g | net carbs: 2g | fiber: 1g

Tomato and Spinach Egg

Prep time: 10 minutes | Cook time: 15 minutes | Serves 4T

2 cups 100% liquid egg whites

3 tablespoons salted butter, melted

¼ teaspoon salt

¼ teaspoon onion powder

½ medium Roma tomato, cored and diced

½ cup chopped fresh spinach leaves

1. In a large bowl, whisk egg whites with butter, salt, and onion powder. Stir in tomato and spinach, then pour evenly into four 4-inch ramekins greased with cooking spray.
2. Place ramekins into air fryer basket. Adjust the temperature to 300°F (150ºC) and set the timer for 15 minutes. Eggs will be fully cooked and firm in the center when done. Serve warm.

Per Serving

calories: 146 | fat: 8g | protein: 14g | carbs: 1g | net carbs: 1g | fiber: 0g

Sausage Egg Cup

Prep time: 10 minutes | Cook time: 15 minutes | Serves 6

12 ounces (340 g) ground pork breakfast sausage

6 large eggs

½ teaspoon salt

¼ teaspoon ground black pepper

½ teaspoon crushed red pepper flakes

1. Place sausage in six 4-inch ramekins (about 2 ounces (57 g) per ramekin) greased with cooking oil. Press sausage down to cover bottom and about ½-inch up the sides of ramekins. Crack one egg into each ramekin and sprinkle evenly with salt, black pepper, and red pepper flakes.
2. Place ramekins into air fryer basket. Adjust the temperature to 350°F (180ºC) and set the timer for 15 minutes. Egg cups will be done when sausage is fully cooked to at least 145°F (63ºC) and the egg is firm. Serve warm.

Per Serving

calories: 267 | fat: 21g | protein: 14g | carbs: 1g | net carbs: 1g | fiber: 0g

Cheesy Ham Egg

Prep time: 10 minutes | Cook time: 15 minutes | Serves 4

4 medium green bell peppers, tops removed, seeded

1 tablespoon coconut oil

3 ounces (85 g) chopped cooked no-sugar-added ham

¼ cup peeled and chopped white onion

4 large eggs

½ teaspoon salt

1 cup shredded mild Cheddar cheese

1. Place peppers upright into ungreased air fryer basket. Drizzle each pepper with coconut oil. Divide ham and onion evenly among peppers.
2. In a medium bowl, whisk eggs, then sprinkle with salt. Pour mixture evenly into each pepper. Top each with ¼ cup Cheddar.
3. Adjust the temperature to 320°F (160°C) and set the timer for 15 minutes. Peppers will be tender and eggs will be firm when done.
4. Serve warm on four medium plates.

Per Serving

calories: 281 | fat: 18g | protein: 18g | carbs: 8g | net carbs: 6g | fiber: 2g

Cheesy Roll

Prep time: 10 minutes | Cook time: 20 minutes | Makes 12 rolls

2½ cups shredded Mozzarella cheese

2 ounces (57 g) cream cheese, softened

1 cup blanched finely ground almond flour

½ teaspoon vanilla extract

½ cup erythritol

1 tablespoon ground cinnamon

1. In a large microwave-safe bowl, combine Mozzarella cheese, cream cheese, and flour. Microwave the mixture on high 90 seconds until cheese is melted.
2. Add vanilla extract and erythritol, and mix 2 minutes until a dough forms.
3. Once the dough is cool enough to work with your hands, about 2 minutes, spread it out into a 12-inch × 4-inch rectangle on ungreased parchment paper. Evenly sprinkle dough with cinnamon.
4. Starting at the long side of the dough, roll lengthwise to form a log. Slice the log into twelve even pieces.
5. Divide rolls between two ungreased 6-inch round nonstick baking dishes. Place one dish into air fryer basket. Adjust the temperature to 375°F (190°C) and set the timer for 10 minutes.
6. Cinnamon rolls will be done when golden around the edges and mostly firm. Repeat with second dish. Allow rolls to cool in dishes 10 minutes before serving.

Per Serving

calories: 145 | fat: 10g | protein: 8g | carbs: 10g | net carbs: 9g | fiber: 1g

Cheesy Omelet

Prep time: 5 minutes | Cook time: 12 minutes | Serves 2

4 large eggs

1½ cups chopped fresh spinach leaves

2 tablespoons peeled and chopped yellow onion

2 tablespoons salted butter, melted

½ cup shredded mild Cheddar cheese

¼ teaspoon salt

1. In an ungreased 6-inch round nonstick baking dish, whisk eggs. Stir in spinach, onion, butter, Cheddar, and salt.
2. Place dish into air fryer basket. Adjust the temperature to 320°F (160°C) and set the timer for 12 minutes. Omelet will be done when browned on the top and firm in the middle.
3. Slice in half and serve warm on two medium plates.

Per Serving

calories: 368 | fat: 28g | protein: 20g | carbs: 3g | net carbs:2g | fiber: 1g

Air Fried Cheese Soufflés

Prep time: 15 minutes | Cook time: 12 minutes | Serves 4

3 large eggs, whites and yolks separated

¼ teaspoon cream of tartar

½ cup shredded sharp Cheddar cheese

3 ounces (85 g) cream cheese, softened

1. In a large bowl, beat egg whites together with cream of tartar until soft peaks form, about 2 minutes.
2. In a separate medium bowl, beat egg yolks, Cheddar, and cream cheese together until frothy, about 1 minute. Add egg yolk mixture to whites, gently folding until combined.
3. Pour mixture evenly into four 4-inch ramekins greased with cooking spray. Place ramekins into air fryer basket. Adjust the temperature to 350ºF (180ºC) and set the timer for 12 minutes. Eggs will be browned on the top and firm in the center when done. Serve warm.

Per Serving

calories: 183 | fat: 14g | protein: 9g | carbs: 1g | net carbs: 1g | fiber: 0g

Bacon and Cheese Quiche

Prep time: 5 minutes | Cook time: 12 minutes | Serves 2

3 large eggs

2 tablespoons heavy whipping cream

¼ teaspoon salt

4 slices cooked sugar-free bacon, crumbled

½ cup shredded mild Cheddar cheese

1. In a large bowl, whisk eggs, cream, and salt together until combined. Mix in bacon and Cheddar.
2. Pour mixture evenly into two ungreased 4-inch ramekins. Place into air fryer basket. Adjust the temperature to 320°F (160ºC) and set the timer for 12 minutes. Quiche will be fluffy and set in the middle when done.
3. Let quiche cool in ramekins 5 minutes. Serve warm.

Per Serving

calories: 380 | fat: 28g | protein: 24g | carbs: 2g | net carbs: 2g | fiber: 0g

Sausage Cheese Meatball

Prep time: 10 minutes | Cook time: 15 minutes | Serves 18 meatballs

1 pound (454 g) ground pork breakfast sausage

½ teaspoon salt

¼ teaspoon ground black pepper

½ cup shredded sharp Cheddar cheese

1 ounce (28 g) cream cheese, softened

1 large egg, whisked

1. Combine all ingredients in a large bowl. Form mixture into eighteen 1-inch meatballs.
2. Place meatballs into ungreased air fryer basket. Adjust the temperature to 400°F and set the timer for 15 minutes, shaking basket three times during cooking. Meatballs will be browned on the outside and have an internal temperature of at least 145°F (63ºC) when completely cooked. Serve warm.

Per Serving

calories: 288 | fat: 24g | protein: 11g | carbs: 1g | net carbs: 1g | fiber: 0g

Sausage Burger with Avocado

Prep time: 5 minutes | Cook time: 15 minutes | Serves 4

1 pound (454 g) ground turkey breakfast sausage

½ teaspoon salt

¼ teaspoon ground black pepper

¼ cup seeded and chopped green bell pepper

2 tablespoons mayonnaise

1 medium avocado, peeled, pitted, and sliced

1. In a large bowl, mix sausage with salt, black pepper, bell pepper, and mayonnaise. Form meat into four patties.

2. Place patties into ungreased air fryer basket. Adjust the temperature to 370°F and set the timer for 15 minutes, turning patties halfway through cooking. Burgers will be done when dark brown and they have an internal temperature of at least 165°F (74ºC).
3. Serve burgers topped with avocado slices on four medium plates.

Per Serving

calories: 276 | fat: 17g | protein: 22g | carbs: 4g | net carbs: 1g | fiber: 3g

Bacon Cheese Pizza

Prep time: 5 minutes | Cook time: 10 minutes | Serves 2

1 cup shredded Mozzarella cheese

1 ounce (28 g) cream cheese, broken into small pieces

4 slices cooked sugar-free bacon, chopped

¼ cup chopped pickled jalapeños

1 large egg, whisked

¼ teaspoon salt

1. Place Mozzarella in a single layer on the bottom of an ungreased 6-inch round nonstick baking dish. Scatter cream cheese pieces, bacon, and jalapeños over Mozzarella, then pour egg evenly around baking dish.
2. Sprinkle with salt and place into air fryer basket. Adjust the temperature to 330°F (166ºC) and set the timer for 10 minutes. When cheese is brown and egg is set, pizza will be done.
3. Let cool on a large plate 5 minutes before serving.

Per Serving

calories: 361 | fat: 24g | protein: 26g | carbs: 5g | net carbs: 5g | fiber: 0g

Cheesy Pepperoni Egg

Prep time: 5 minutes | Cook time: 10 minutes | Serves 2

1 cup shredded Mozzarella cheese

7 slices pepperoni, chopped

1 large egg, whisked

¼ teaspoon dried oregano

¼ teaspoon dried parsley

¼ teaspoon garlic powder

¼ teaspoon salt

1. Place Mozzarella in a single layer on the bottom of an ungreased 6-inch round nonstick baking dish. Scatter pepperoni over cheese, then pour egg evenly around baking dish.
2. Sprinkle with remaining ingredients and place into air fryer basket. Adjust the temperature to 330°F (166ºC) and set the timer for 10 minutes. When cheese is brown and egg is set, dish will be done.
3. Let cool in dish 5 minutes before serving.

Per Serving

calories: 241 | fat: 15g | protein: 19g | carbs: 4g | net carbs: 4g | fiber: 0g

Pecan Granola

Prep time: 10 minutes | Cook time: 5 minutes | Serves 6

2 cups pecans, chopped

1 cup unsweetened coconut flakes

1 cup almond slivers

$^1/_3$ cup sunflower seeds

¼ cup golden flaxseed

¼ cup low-carb, sugar-free chocolate chips

¼ cup granular erythritol

2 tablespoons unsalted butter

1 teaspoon ground cinnamon

1. In a large bowl, mix all ingredients.

2. Place the mixture into a 4-cup round baking dish. Place dish into the air fryer basket.
3. Adjust the temperature to 320°F (160°C) and set the timer for 5 minutes.
4. Allow to cool completely before serving.

Per Serving

calories: 617 | fat: 55g | protein: 11g | carbs: 32g | net carbs: 21g | fiber: 11g

Broccoli Frittata

Prep time: 15 minutes | Cook time: 12 minutes | Serves 4

6 large eggs

¼ cup heavy whipping cream

½ cup chopped broccoli

¼ cup chopped yellow onion

¼ cup chopped green bell pepper

1. In a large bowl, whisk eggs and heavy whipping cream. Mix in broccoli, onion, and bell pepper.
2. Pour into a 6-inch round oven-safe baking dish. Place baking dish into the air fryer basket.
3. Adjust the temperature to 350°F (180°C) and set the timer for 12 minutes.
4. Eggs should be firm and cooked fully when the frittata is done. Serve warm.

Per Serving

calories: 168 | fat: 11g | protein: 10g | carbs: 3g | net carbs: 2g | fiber: 1g

Lemony Cake

Prep time: 10 minutes | Cook time: 14 minutes | Serves 6

1 cup blanched finely ground almond flour

½ cup powdered erythritol

½ teaspoon baking powder

¼ cup unsalted butter, melted

¼ cup unsweetened almond milk

2 large eggs

1 teaspoon vanilla extract

1 medium lemon

1 teaspoon poppy seeds

1. In a large bowl, mix almond flour, erythritol, baking powder, butter, almond milk, eggs, and vanilla.
2. Slice the lemon in half and squeeze the juice into a small bowl, then add to the batter.
3. Using a fine grater, zest the lemon and add 1 tablespoon zest to the batter and stir. Add poppy seeds to batter.
4. Pour batter into nonstick 6-inch round cake pan. Place pan into the air fryer basket.
5. Adjust the temperature to 300°F (150°C) and set the timer for 14 minutes.
6. When fully cooked, a toothpick inserted in center will come out mostly clean. The cake will finish cooking and firm up as it cools. Serve at room temperature.

Per Serving

calories: 204 | fat: 18g | protein: 6g | carbs: 17g | net carbs: 15g | fiber: 2g

Aromatic Cake

Prep time: 10 minutes | Cook time: 7 minutes | Serves 4

½ cup blanched finely ground almond flour
¼ cup powdered erythritol
½ teaspoon baking powder
2 tablespoons unsalted butter, softened
1 large egg
½ teaspoon unflavored gelatin
½ teaspoon vanilla extract
½ teaspoon ground cinnamon

1. In a large bowl, mix almond flour, erythritol, and baking powder. Add butter, egg, gelatin, vanilla, and cinnamon. Pour into 6-inch round baking pan.
2. Place pan into the air fryer basket.
3. Adjust the temperature to 300°F (150°C) and set the timer for 7 minutes.
4. When the cake is completely cooked, a toothpick will come out clean. Cut cake into four and serve.

Per Serving

calories: 153 | fat: 13g | protein: 5g | carbs: 13g | net carbs: 11g | fiber: 2g

Cheesy Cauliflower Hash Browns

Prep time: 20 minutes | Cook time: 12 minutes | Serves 4

1 (12-ounce / 340-g) steamer bag cauliflower

1 large egg

1 cup shredded sharp Cheddar cheese

1. Place bag in microwave and cook according to package instructions. Allow to cool completely and put cauliflower into a cheesecloth or kitchen towel and squeeze to remove excess moisture.
2. Mash cauliflower with a fork and add egg and cheese.
3. Cut a piece of parchment to fit your air fryer basket. Take ¼ of the mixture and form it into a hash brown patty shape. Place it onto the parchment and into the air fryer basket, working in batches if necessary.
4. Adjust the temperature to 400°F (205ºC) and set the timer for 12 minutes.
5. Flip the hash browns halfway through the cooking time. When completely cooked, they will be golden brown. Serve immediately.

Per Serving

calories: 153 | fat: 9g | protein: 10g | carbs: 5g | net carbs: 3g | fiber: 2g

Cheesy Sausage Pepper

Prep time: 15 minutes | Cook time: 15 minutes | Serves 4

½ pound (227 g) spicy ground pork breakfast sausage

4 large eggs

4 ounces (113 g) full-fat cream cheese, softened

¼ cup canned diced tomatoes and green chiles, drained

4 large poblano peppers

8 tablespoons shredded pepper jack cheese

½ cup full-fat sour cream

1. In a medium skillet over medium heat, crumble and brown the ground sausage until no pink remains. Remove sausage and drain the fat from the pan. Crack eggs into the pan, scramble, and cook until no longer runny.
2. Place cooked sausage in a large bowl and fold in cream cheese. Mix in diced tomatoes and chiles. Gently fold in eggs.

3. Cut a 4-inch–5-inch slit in the top of each poblano, removing the seeds and white membrane with a small knife. Separate the filling into four servings and spoon carefully into each pepper. Top each with 2 tablespoons pepper jack cheese.
4. Place each pepper into the air fryer basket.
5. Adjust the temperature to 350°F (180°C) and set the timer for 15 minutes.
6. Peppers will be soft and cheese will be browned when ready. Serve immediately with sour cream on top.

Per Serving

calories: 489 | fat: 35g | protein: 23g | carbs: 13g | net carbs: 9g | fiber: 4g

Cheesy Egg

Prep time: 5 minutes | Cook time: 15 minutes | Serves 2

4 large eggs

2 tablespoons unsalted butter, melted

½ cup shredded sharp Cheddar cheese

1. Crack eggs into 2-cup round baking dish and whisk. Place dish into the air fryer basket.
2. Adjust the temperature to 400°F (205°C) and set the timer for 10 minutes.
3. After 5 minutes, stir the eggs and add the butter and cheese. Let cook 3 more minutes and stir again.
4. Allow eggs to finish cooking an additional 2 minutes or remove if they are to your desired liking.
5. Use a fork to fluff. Serve warm.

Per Serving

calories: 359 | fat: 27g | protein: 20g | carbs: 1g | net carbs: 1g | fiber: 0g

Bacon Cheese Egg with Avocado

Prep time: 15 minutes | Cook time: 20 minutes | Serves 4

6 large eggs

¼ cup heavy whipping cream

1½ cups chopped cauliflower

1 cup shredded medium Cheddar cheese

1 medium avocado, peeled and pitted

8 tablespoons full-fat sour cream

2 scallions, sliced on the bias

12 slices sugar-free bacon, cooked and crumbled

1. In a medium bowl, whisk eggs and cream together. Pour into a 4-cup round baking dish.
2. Add cauliflower and mix, then top with Cheddar. Place dish into the air fryer basket.
3. Adjust the temperature to 320°F (160°C) and set the timer for 20 minutes.
4. When completely cooked, eggs will be firm and cheese will be browned. Slice into four pieces.
5. Slice avocado and divide evenly among pieces. Top each piece with 2 tablespoons sour cream, sliced scallions, and crumbled bacon.

Per Serving

calories: 512 | fat: 38g | protein: 27g | carbs: 8g | net carbs: 5g | fiber: 3g

Cheesy Avocado Cauliflower

Prep time: 15 minutes | Cook time: 8 minutes | Serves 2

1 (12-ounce / 340-g) steamer bag cauliflower

1 large egg

½ cup shredded Mozzarella cheese

1 ripe medium avocado

½ teaspoon garlic powder

¼ teaspoon ground black pepper

1. Cook cauliflower according to package instructions. Remove from bag and place into cheesecloth or clean towel to remove excess moisture.
2. Place cauliflower into a large bowl and mix in egg and Mozzarella. Cut a piece of parchment to fit your air fryer basket. Separate the cauliflower mixture into two, and place it on the parchment in two mounds. Press out the cauliflower mounds into a ¼-inch-thick rectangle. Place the parchment into the air fryer basket.
3. Adjust the temperature to 400°F (205°C) and set the timer for 8 minutes.
4. Flip the cauliflower halfway through the cooking time.
5. When the timer beeps, remove the parchment and allow the cauliflower to cool 5 minutes.

6. Cut open the avocado and remove the pit. Scoop out the inside, place it in a medium bowl, and mash it with garlic powder and pepper. Spread onto the cauliflower. Serve immediately.

Per Serving

calories: 278 | fat: 15g | protein: 14g | carbs: 16g | net carbs: 8g | fiber: 8g

Air Fried Spaghetti Squash

Prep time: 15 minutes | Cook time: 8 minutes | Serves 4

2 cups cooked spaghetti squash

2 tablespoons unsalted butter, softened

1 large egg

¼ cup blanched finely ground almond flour

2 stalks green onion, sliced

½ teaspoon garlic powder

1 teaspoon dried parsley

1. Remove excess moisture from the squash using a cheesecloth or kitchen towel.
2. Mix all ingredients in a large bowl. Form into four patties.
3. Cut a piece of parchment to fit your air fryer basket. Place each patty on the parchment and place into the air fryer basket.
4. Adjust the temperature to 400°F (205°C) and set the timer for 8 minutes.
5. Flip the patties halfway through the cooking time. Serve warm.

Per Serving

calories: 131 | fat: 10g | protein: 4g | carbs: 7g | net carbs: 5g | fiber: 2g

Lettuce Wrap with Bacon

Prep time: 20 minutes | Cook time: 13 minutes | Serves 4

8 ounces (227 g) (about 12 slices) reduced-sodium bacon

8 tablespoons mayonnaise

8 large romaine lettuce leaves

4 Roma tomatoes, sliced

Salt and freshly ground black pepper

1. Arrange the bacon in a single layer in the air fryer basket. (It's OK if the bacon sits a bit on the sides.) Set the air fryer to 350°F (180°C) and cook for 10 minutes. Check for crispiness and cook for 2 to 3 minutes longer if needed. Cook in batches, if necessary, and drain the grease in between batches.
2. Spread 1 tablespoon of mayonnaise on each of the lettuce leaves and top with the tomatoes and cooked bacon. Season to taste with salt and freshly ground black pepper. Roll the lettuce leaves as you would a burrito, securing with a toothpick if desired.

Per Serving

calories: 370 | fat: 34g | protein: 11g | carbs: 7g | net carbs: 4g | fiber: 3g

Pork Sausage Eggs With Mustard Sauce

Prep time: 20 minutes | Cook time: 12 minutes | Serves 8

1 pound (454 g) pork sausage

8 soft-boiled or hard-boiled eggs, peeled

1 large egg

2 tablespoons milk

1 cup crushed pork rinds

Smoky Mustard Sauce:

¼ cup mayonnaise

2 tablespoons sour cream

1 tablespoon Dijon mustard

1 teaspoon chipotle hot sauce

1. Preheat the air fryer to 390°F (199°C).
2. Divide the sausage into 8 portions. Take each portion of sausage, pat it down into a patty, and place 1 egg in the middle, gently wrapping the sausage around the egg until the egg is completely covered. (Wet your hands slightly if you find the sausage to be too sticky.) Repeat with the remaining eggs and sausage.
3. In a small shallow bowl, whisk the egg and milk until frothy. In another shallow bowl, place the crushed pork rinds. Working one at a time, dip a sausage-wrapped egg into the beaten egg and then into the pork rinds, gently rolling to coat evenly. Repeat with the remaining sausage-wrapped eggs.

4. Arrange the eggs in a single layer in the air fryer basket, and lightly spray with olive oil. Air fry for 10 to 12 minutes, pausing halfway through the baking time to turn the eggs, until the eggs are hot and the sausage is cooked through.
5. To make the sauce: In a small bowl, combine the mayonnaise, sour cream, Dijon, and hot sauce. Whisk until thoroughly combined. Serve with the Scotch eggs.

Per Serving

calories: 340 | fat: 28g | protein: 22g | carbs: 1g | net carbs: 1g | fiber: 0g

Air Fried Mushroon with Tomato

Prep time: 15 minutes | Cook time: 14 minutes | Serves 2

1 tablespoon olive oil

2 cloves garlic, minced

¼ teaspoon dried thyme

2 portobello mushrooms, stems removed and gills scraped out

2 Roma tomatoes, halved lengthwise

Salt and freshly ground black pepper

2 large eggs

2 tablespoons grated Pecorino Romano cheese

1 tablespoon chopped fresh parsley, for garnish

1. Preheat the air fryer to 400°F (205°C).
2. In a small bowl, combine the olive oil, garlic, and thyme. Brush the mixture over the mushrooms and tomatoes until thoroughly coated. Season to taste with salt and freshly ground black pepper.
3. Arrange the vegetables, cut side up, in the air fryer basket. Crack an egg into the center of each mushroom and sprinkle with cheese. Air fry for 10 to 14 minutes until the vegetables are tender and the whites are firm. When cool enough to handle, coarsely chop the tomatoes and place on top of the eggs. Scatter parsley on top just before serving.

Per Serving

calories: 255 | fat: 20g | protein: 11g | carbs: 10g | net carbs: 7g | fiber: 3g

Mushroom Frittata

Prep time: 15 minutes | Cook time: 20 minutes | Serves 2

1 tablespoon olive oil

1½ cups broccoli florets, finely chopped

½ cup sliced brown mushrooms

¼ cup finely chopped onion

½ teaspoon salt

¼ teaspoon freshly ground black pepper

6 eggs

¼ cup Parmesan cheese

1. In an 8-inch nonstick cake pan, combine the olive oil, broccoli, mushrooms, onion, salt, and pepper. Stir until the vegetables are thoroughly coated with oil. Place the cake pan in the air fryer basket and set the air fryer to 400°F (205ºC). Air fry for 5 minutes until the vegetables soften.
2. Meanwhile, in a medium bowl, whisk the eggs and Parmesan until thoroughly combined. Pour the egg mixture into the pan and shake gently to distribute the vegetables. Air fry for another 15 minutes until the eggs are set.
3. Remove from the air fryer and let sit for 5 minutes to cool slightly. Use a silicone spatula to gently lift the frittata onto a plate before serving.

Per Serving

calories: 360 | fat: 25g | protein: 25g | carbs: 10g | net carbs: 8g | fiber: 2g

Turkey Sausage

Prep time: 15 minutes | Cook time: 20 minutes | Serves 8

1½ pounds (680g) 85% lean ground turkey

3 cloves garlic, finely chopped

¼ onion, grated

1 teaspoon Tabasco sauce

1 teaspoon Creole seasoning

1 teaspoon dried thyme

½ teaspoon paprika

½ teaspoon cayenne

1. Preheat the air fryer to 370°F (188°C).
2. In a large bowl, combine the turkey, garlic, onion, Tabasco, Creole seasoning, thyme, paprika, and cayenne. Mix with clean hands until thoroughly combined. Shape into 16 patties, about ½ -inch thick. (Wet your hands slightly if you find the sausage too sticky to handle.)
3. Working in batches if necessary, arrange the patties in a single layer in the air fryer basket. Pausing halfway through the cooking time to flip the patties, air fry for 15 to 20 minutes until a thermometer inserted into the thickest portion registers 165°F (74°C).

Per Serving

calories: 170 | fat: 11g | protein: 16g | carbs: 1g | net carbs: 1g | fiber: 0g

Appetizers and Snacks

Cauliflower with Buffalo Sauce

Prep time: 5 minutes | Cook time: 15 minutes | Serves 6

1 medium head cauliflower, leaves and core removed, cut into bite-sized pieces

4 tablespoons salted butter, melted

¼ cup dry ranch seasoning

$^1/_3$ cup sugar-free buffalo sauce

1. Place cauliflower pieces into a large bowl. Pour butter over cauliflower and toss to coat. Sprinkle in ranch seasoning and toss to coat.
2. Place cauliflower into ungreased air fryer basket. Adjust the temperature to 350°F (180ºC) and set the timer for 12 minutes, shaking the basket three times during cooking.
3. When timer beeps, place cooked cauliflower in a clean large bowl. Toss with buffalo sauce, then return to air fryer basket to cook another 3 minutes. Cauliflower bites will be darkened at the edges and tender when done. Serve warm.

Per Serving

calories: 112 | fat: 7g | protein: 2g | carbs: 9g | net carbs: 7g | fiber: 2g

Cheesy Bacon-Wrapped Jalapeño

Prep time: 10 minutes | Cook time: 12 minutes | Makes 12 poppers

3 ounces (85 g) cream cheese, softened

$^1/_3$ cup shredded mild Cheddar cheese

¼ teaspoon garlic powder

6 jalapeños (approximately 4-inch long), tops removed, sliced in half lengthwise and seeded

12 slices sugar-free bacon

1. Place cream cheese, Cheddar, and garlic powder in a large microwave-safe bowl. Microwave 30 seconds on high, then stir. Spoon cheese mixture evenly into hollowed jalapeños.
2. Wrap 1 slice bacon around each jalapeño half, completely covering jalapeño, and secure with a toothpick. Place jalapeños into ungreased air fryer basket. Adjust the temperature to 400°F (205ºC) and set the timer for 12 minutes, turning jalapeños halfway through cooking. Bacon will be crispy when done. Serve warm.

Per Serving

calories: 278 | fat: 21g | protein: 15g | carbs: 3g | net carbs: 2g | fiber: 1g

Prosciutto Cheese Asparagus Roll

Prep time: 10 minutes | Cook time: 10 minutes | Serves 4

1 pound (454 g) asparagus

12 (0.5-ounce 14-g) slices prosciutto

1 tablespoon coconut oil, melted

2 teaspoons lemon juice

⅛ teaspoon red pepper flakes

⅓ cup grated Parmesan cheese

2 tablespoons salted butter, melted

1. On a clean work surface, place an asparagus spear onto a slice of prosciutto.
2. Drizzle with coconut oil and lemon juice. Sprinkle red pepper flakes and Parmesan across asparagus. Roll prosciutto around asparagus spear. Place into the air fryer basket.
3. Adjust the temperature to 375°F (190°C) and set the timer for 10 minutes.
4. Drizzle the asparagus roll with butter before serving.

Per Serving

calories: 263 | fat: 20g | protein: 14g | carbs: 7g | net carbs: 4g | fiber: 3g

Cheesy Mushroom

Prep time: 10 minutes | Cook time: 8 minutes | Serves 20 mushrooms

4 ounces (113 g) cream cheese, softened

6 tablespoons shredded pepper jack cheese

2 tablespoons chopped pickled jalapeños

20 medium button mushrooms, stems removed

2 tablespoons olive oil

¼ teaspoon salt

⅛ teaspoon ground black pepper

1. In a large bowl, mix cream cheese, pepper jack, and jalapeños together.
2. Drizzle mushrooms with olive oil, then sprinkle with salt and pepper. Spoon 2 tablespoons cheese mixture into each mushroom and place in a single layer into ungreased air fryer basket. Adjust the temperature to 370°F (188ºC) and set the timer for 8 minutes, checking halfway through cooking to ensure even cooking, rearranging if some are darker than others. When they're golden and cheese is bubbling, mushrooms will be done. Serve warm.

Per Serving

calories: 87 | fat: 7g | protein: 3g | carbs: 2g | net carbs: 2g | fiber: 0g

Three Cheese Dip

Prep time: 5 minutes | Cook time: 12 minutes | Serves 8

8 ounces (227 g) cream cheese, softened
½ cup mayonnaise
¼ cup sour cream
½ cup shredded sharp Cheddar cheese
¼ cup shredded Monterey jack cheese

1. In a large bowl, combine all ingredients. Scoop mixture into an ungreased 4-cup nonstick baking dish and place into air fryer basket.
2. Adjust the temperature to 375°F (190ºC) and set the timer for 12 minutes. Dip will be browned on top and bubbling when done. Serve warm.

Per Serving

calories: 245 | fat: 23g | protein: 5g | carbs: 2g | net carbs: 2g | fiber: 0g

Cheese Chicken Dip

Prep time: 10 minutes | Cook time: 12 minutes | Serves 8

8 ounces (227 g) cream cheese, softened
2 cups chopped cooked chicken thighs
½ cup sugar-free buffalo sauce

1 cup shredded mild Cheddar cheese, divided

1. In a large bowl, combine cream cheese, chicken, buffalo sauce, and ½ cup Cheddar. Scoop dip into an ungreased 4-cup nonstick baking dish and top with remaining Cheddar.
2. Place dish into air fryer basket. Adjust the temperature to 375°F (190ºC) and set the timer for 12 minutes. Dip will be browned on top and bubbling when done. Serve warm.

Per Serving

calories: 222 | fat: 15g | protein: 14g | carbs:1g | net carbs: 1g | fiber: 0g

Beef and Bacon Cheese Dip

Prep time: 20 minutes | Cook time: 10 minutes | Serves 6

8 ounces (227 g) full-fat cream cheese

¼ cup full-fat mayonnaise

¼ cup full-fat sour cream

¼ cup chopped onion

1 teaspoon garlic powder

1 tablespoon Worcestershire sauce

1¼ cups shredded medium Cheddar cheese, divided

½ pound (227g) cooked 80/20 ground beef

6 slices sugar-free bacon, cooked and crumbled

2 large pickle spears, chopped

1. Place cream cheese in a large microwave-safe bowl and microwave for 45 seconds. Stir in mayonnaise, sour cream, onion, garlic powder, Worcestershire sauce, and 1 cup Cheddar. Add cooked ground beef and bacon. Sprinkle remaining Cheddar on top.
2. Place in 6-inch bowl and put into the air fryer basket.
3. Adjust the temperature to 400°F (205ºC) and set the timer for 10 minutes.
4. Dip is done when top is golden and bubbling. Sprinkle pickles over dish. Serve warm.

Per Serving

calories: 457 | fat: 35g | protein: 22g | carbs: 4g | net carbs: 3g | fiber: 1g

Cheesy Spinach Artichoke Dip

Prep time: 10 minutes | Cook time: 10 minutes | Serves 6

10 ounces (283 g) frozen spinach, drained and thawed

1 (14-ounce / 397-g) can artichoke hearts, drained and chopped

¼ cup chopped pickled jalapeños

8 ounces (227 g) full-fat cream cheese, softened

¼ cup full-fat mayonnaise

¼ cup full-fat sour cream

½ teaspoon garlic powder

¼ cup grated Parmesan cheese

1 cup shredded pepper jack cheese

1. Mix all ingredients in a 4-cup baking bowl. Place into the air fryer basket.
2. Adjust the temperature to 320°F (160°C) and set the timer for 10 minutes.
3. Remove when brown and bubbling. Serve warm.

Per Serving

calories: 226 | fat: 15g | protein: 10g | carbs: 10g | net carbs: 6g | fiber: 4g

Cheesy Pizza Crust

Prep time: 5 minutes | Cook time: 10 minutes | Serves 1

½ cup shredded whole-milk Mozzarella cheese

2 tablespoons blanched finely ground almond flour

1 tablespoon full-fat cream cheese

1 large egg white

1. Place Mozzarella, almond flour, and cream cheese in a medium microwave-safe bowl. Microwave for 30 seconds. Stir until smooth ball of dough forms. Add egg white and stir until soft round dough forms.
2. Press into a 6-inch round pizza crust.
3. Cut a piece of parchment to fit your air fryer basket and place crust on parchment. Place into the air fryer basket.
4. Adjust the temperature to 350°F (180°C) and set the timer for 10 minutes.

5. Flip after 5 minutes and at this time place any desired toppings on the crust. Continue cooking until golden. Serve immediately.

Per Serving

calories: 314 | fat: 22g | protein: 20g | carbs: 5g | net carbs: 3g | fiber: 2g

Sausage and Bacon Cheese Pizza

Prep time: 5 minutes | Cook time: 5 minutes | Serves 1

½ cup shredded Mozzarella cheese

7 slices pepperoni

¼ cup cooked ground sausage

2 slices sugar-free bacon, cooked and crumbled

1 tablespoon grated Parmesan cheese

2 tablespoons low-carb, sugar-free pizza sauce, for dipping

1. Cover the bottom of a 6-inch cake pan with Mozzarella. Place pepperoni, sausage, and bacon on top of cheese and sprinkle with Parmesan. Place pan into the air fryer basket.
2. Adjust the temperature to 400°F (205°C) and set the timer for 5 minutes.
3. Remove when cheese is bubbling and golden. Serve warm with pizza sauce for dipping.

Per Serving

calories: 466 | fat: 34g | protein: 28g | carbs: 5g | net carbs: 4g | fiber: 1g

Air Fried Almond

Prep time: 5 minutes | Cook time: 6 minutes | Serves 4

1 cup raw almonds

2 teaspoons coconut oil

1 teaspoon chili powder

¼ teaspoon cumin

¼ teaspoon smoked paprika

¼ teaspoon onion powder

1. In a large bowl, toss all ingredients until almonds are evenly coated with oil and spices. Place almonds into the air fryer basket.
2. Adjust the temperature to 320°F (160ºC) and set the timer for 6 minutes.
3. Toss the fryer basket halfway through the cooking time. Allow to cool completely.

Per Serving

calories: 182 | fat: 16g | protein: 6g | carbs: 7g | net carbs: 3g | fiber: 4g

Cheesy Chicken with Bacon

Prep time: 10 minutes | Cook time: 15 minutes | Serves 6

2 (6-ounce / 170-g) boneless, skinless chicken breasts, cut into 1-inch cubes

1 tablespoon coconut oil

½ teaspoon salt

¼ teaspoon ground black pepper

1/3 cup ranch dressing

½ cup shredded Colby cheese

4 slices cooked sugar-free bacon, crumbled

1. Drizzle chicken with coconut oil. Sprinkle with salt and pepper, and place into an ungreased 6-inch round nonstick baking dish.
2. Place dish into air fryer basket. Adjust the temperature to 370°F (188ºC) and set the timer for 10 minutes, stirring chicken halfway through cooking.
3. When timer beeps, drizzle ranch dressing over chicken and top with Colby and bacon. Adjust the temperature to 400°F (205ºC) and set the timer for 5 minutes. When done, chicken will be browned and have an internal temperature of at least 165°F (74ºC). Serve warm.

Per Serving

calories: 164 | fat: 9g | protein: 18g | carbs: 0g | net carbs: 0g | fiber: 0g

Beef Jerky

Prep time: 5 minutes | Cook time: 4 hours | Serves 10

1 pound (454 g) flat iron beef, thinly sliced

¼ cup coconut aminos

2 teaspoons Worcestershire sauce

¼ teaspoon crushed red pepper flakes

¼ teaspoon garlic powder

¼ teaspoon onion powder

1. Place all ingredients into a plastic storage bag or covered container and marinate 2 hours in refrigerator.
2. Place each slice of jerky on the air fryer rack in a single layer.
3. Adjust the temperature to 160°F (71ºC) and set the timer for 4 hours.
4. Cool and store in airtight container up to 1 week.

Per Serving

calories: 85 | fat: 3g | protein: 10g | carbs: 1g | net carbs: 1g | fiber: 0g

Pepperoni Cheese Roll

Prep time: 5 minutes | Cook time: 8 minutes | Makes 12 rolls

2½ cups shredded Mozzarella cheese

2 ounces (57 g) cream cheese, softened

1 cup blanched finely ground almond flour

48 slices pepperoni

2 teaspoons Italian seasoning

1. In a large microwave-safe bowl, combine Mozzarella, cream cheese, and flour. Microwave on high 90 seconds until cheese is melted.
2. Using a wooden spoon, mix melted mixture 2 minutes until a dough forms.
3. Once dough is cool enough to work with your hands, about 2 minutes, spread it out into a 12-inch × 4-inch rectangle on ungreased parchment paper. Line dough with pepperoni, divided into four even rows. Sprinkle Italian seasoning evenly over pepperoni.

4. Starting at the long end of the dough, roll up until a log is formed. Slice the log into twelve even pieces.
5. Place pizza rolls in an ungreased 6-inch nonstick baking dish. Adjust the temperature to 375°F (190°C) and set the timer for 8 minutes. Rolls will be golden and firm when done. Allow cooked rolls to cool 10 minutes before serving.

Per Serving

calories: 366 | fat: 27g | protein: 20g | carbs: 7g | net carbs: 5g | fiber: 2g

Spinach Turkey Meatball

Prep time: 10 minutes | Cook time: 10 minutes | Makes 36 meatballs

1 cup fresh spinach leaves
¼ cup peeled and diced red onion
½ cup crumbled feta cheese
1 pound (454 g) 85/15 ground turkey
½ teaspoon salt
½ teaspoon ground cumin
¼ teaspoon ground black pepper

1. Place spinach, onion, and feta in a food processor, and pulse ten times until spinach is chopped. Scoop into a large bowl.
2. Add turkey to bowl and sprinkle with salt, cumin, and pepper. Mix until fully combined. Roll mixture into thirty-six meatballs (about 1 tablespoon each).
3. Place meatballs into ungreased air fryer basket, working in batches if needed. Adjust the temperature to 350°F (180°C) and set the timer for 10 minutes, shaking basket twice during cooking. Meatballs will be browned and have an internal temperature of at least 165°F (74°C) when done. Serve warm.

Per Serving

calories: 115 | fat: 7g | protein: 10g | carbs: 1g | net carbs: 1g | fiber: 0g

Cheesy Calamari Rings

Prep time: 10 minutes | Cook time: 15 minutes | Serves 4

2 large egg yolks

1 cup powdered Parmesan cheese (or pork dust for dairy-free; see [here](#))

¼ cup coconut flour

3 teaspoons dried oregano leaves

½ teaspoon garlic powder

½ teaspoon onion powder

1 pound (454 g) calamari, sliced into rings

Fresh oregano leaves, for garnish (optional)

1 cup no-sugar-added marinara sauce, for serving (optional)

Lemon slices, for serving (optional)

1. Spray the air fryer basket with avocado oil. Preheat the air fryer to 400°F (205ºC).
2. In a shallow dish, whisk the egg yolks. In a separate bowl, mix together the Parmesan, coconut flour, and spices.
3. Dip the calamari rings in the egg yolks, tap off any excess egg, then dip them into the cheese mixture and coat well. Use your hands to press the coating onto the calamari if necessary. Spray the coated rings with avocado oil.
4. Place the calamari rings in the air fryer, leaving space between them, and cook for 15 minutes, or until golden brown. Garnish with fresh oregano, if desired, and serve with marinara sauce for dipping and lemon slices, if desired.
5. Best served fresh. Store leftovers in an airtight container in the fridge for up to 5 days. Reheat in a preheated 400°F (205ºC) air fryer for 3 minutes, or until heated through.

Per Serving

calories: 287 | fat: 13g | protein: 28g | carbs: 11g | net carbs: 8g | fiber: 3g

Bacon-Wrapped Onion Rings

Prep time: 5 minutes | Cook time: 10 minutes | Serves 8

1 large white onion, peeled and cut into 16 (¼-inch-thick) slices

8 slices sugar-free bacon

1. Stack 2 slices onion and wrap with 1 slice bacon. Secure with a toothpick. Repeat with remaining onion slices and bacon.
2. Place onion rings into ungreased air fryer basket. Adjust the temperature to 350°F (180ºC) and set the timer for 10 minutes, turning rings halfway through cooking. Bacon will be crispy when done. Serve warm.

Per Serving

calories: 84 | fat: 4g | protein: 5g | carbs: 8g | net carbs: 6g | fiber: 2g

Bacon-Wrapped Cabbage Bites

Prep time: 10 minutes | Cook time: 12 minutes | Serves 6

3 tablespoons sriracha hot chili sauce, divided

1 medium head cabbage, cored and cut into 12 bite-sized pieces

2 tablespoons coconut oil, melted

½ teaspoon salt

12 slices sugar-free bacon

½ cup mayonnaise

¼ teaspoon garlic powder

1. Evenly brush 2 tablespoons sriracha onto cabbage pieces. Drizzle evenly with coconut oil, then sprinkle with salt.
2. Wrap each cabbage piece with bacon and secure with a toothpick. Place into ungreased air fryer basket. Adjust the temperature to 375°F (190ºC) and set the timer for 12 minutes, turning cabbage halfway through cooking. Bacon will be cooked and crispy when done.
3. In a small bowl, whisk together mayonnaise, garlic powder, and remaining sriracha. Use as a dipping sauce for cabbage bites.

Per Serving

calories: 316 | fat: 26g | protein: 10g | carbs: 11g | net carbs: 7g | fiber: 4g

Cheesy Chicken Wings

Prep time: 5 minutes | Cook time: 25 minutes | Serves 4

2 pounds (907 g) raw chicken wings

1 teaspoon pink Himalayan salt

½ teaspoon garlic powder

1 tablespoon baking powder

4 tablespoons unsalted butter, melted

$1/3$ cup grated Parmesan cheese

¼ teaspoon dried parsley

1. In a large bowl, place chicken wings, salt, ½ teaspoon garlic powder, and baking powder, then toss. Place wings into the air fryer basket.
2. Adjust the temperature to 400°F (205°C) and set the timer for 25 minutes.
3. Toss the basket two or three times during the cooking time.
4. In a small bowl, combine butter, Parmesan, and parsley.
5. Remove wings from the fryer and place into a clean large bowl. Pour the butter mixture over the wings and toss until coated. Serve warm.

Per Serving

calories: 565 | fat: 42g | protein: 42g | carbs: 2g | net carbs: 2g | fiber: 0g

Air Fried Chicken Wings

Prep time: 5 minutes | Cook time: 32 minutes | Serves 1 dozen wings

1 dozen chicken wings or drummies

1 tablespoon coconut oil or bacon fat, melted

2 teaspoons berbere spice

1 teaspoon fine sea salt

**For Serving
(Omit For Egg-Free):**

2 hard-boiled eggs

½ teaspoon fine sea salt

¼ teaspoon berbere spice

¼ teaspoon dried chives

1. Spray the air fryer basket with avocado oil. Preheat the air fryer to 380°F (193ºC).
2. Place the chicken wings in a large bowl. Pour the oil over them and turn to coat completely. Sprinkle the berbere and salt on all sides of the chicken.
3. Place the chicken wings in the air fryer and cook for 25 minutes, flipping after 15 minutes.
4. After 25 minutes, increase the temperature to 400°F (205ºC) and cook for 6 to 7 minutes more, until the skin is browned and crisp.
5. While the chicken cooks, prepare the hard-boiled eggs (if using): Peel the eggs, slice them in half, and season them with the salt, berbere, and dried chives. Serve the chicken and eggs together.
6. Store leftovers in an airtight container in the fridge for up to 4 days. Reheat the chicken in a preheated 400°F (205ºC) air fryer for 5 minutes, or until heated through.

Per Serving

calories: 317 | fat: 24g | protein: 24g | carbs: 1g | net carbs: 1g | fiber: 0g

Golden Pork Egg

Prep time: 10 minutes | Cook time: 25 minutes | Makes 12 eggs

7 large eggs, divided

1 ounce (28 g) plain pork rinds, finely crushed

2 tablespoons mayonnaise

¼ teaspoon salt

¼ teaspoon ground black pepper

1. Place 6 whole eggs into ungreased air fryer basket. Adjust the temperature to 220°F (104ºC) and set the timer for 20 minutes. When done, place eggs into a bowl of ice water to cool 5 minutes.
2. Peel cool eggs, then cut in half lengthwise. Remove yolks and place aside in a medium bowl.
3. In a separate small bowl, whisk remaining raw egg. Place pork rinds in a separate medium bowl. Dip each egg white into whisked egg, then gently coat with pork rinds. Spritz with cooking spray and place into ungreased air fryer basket. Adjust the temperature to 400°F (205ºC) and set the timer for 5 minutes, turning eggs halfway through cooking. Eggs will be golden when done.
4. Mash yolks in bowl with mayonnaise until smooth. Sprinkle with salt and pepper and mix.
5. Spoon 2 tablespoons yolk mixture into each fried egg white. Serve warm.

Per Serving

calories: 141 | fat: 10g | protein: 10g | carbs: 1g | net carbs: 1g | fiber: 0g

Bacon Jalapeño Cheese Bread

Prep time: 10 minutes | Cook time: 15 minutes | Serves 8 sticks

2 cups shredded Mozzarella cheese

¼ cup grated Parmesan cheese

¼ cup chopped pickled jalapeños

2 large eggs

4 slices sugar-free bacon, cooked and chopped

1. Mix all ingredients in a large bowl. Cut a piece of parchment to fit your air fryer basket.
2. Dampen your hands with a bit of water and press out the mixture into a circle. You may need to separate this into two smaller cheese breads, depending on the size of your fryer.
3. Place the parchment and cheese bread into the air fryer basket.
4. Adjust the temperature to 320°F (160°C) and set the timer for 15 minutes.
5. Carefully flip the bread when 5 minutes remain.
6. When fully cooked, the top will be golden brown. Serve warm.

Per Serving

calories: 273 | fat: 18g | protein: 20g | carbs: 3g | net carbs: 2g | fiber: 1g

Cheesy Bacon Pepper

Prep time: 15 minutes | Cook time: 8 minutes | Serves 16 halves

8 mini sweet peppers

4 ounces (113 g) full-fat cream cheese, softened

4 slices sugar-free bacon, cooked and crumbled

¼ cup shredded pepper jack cheese

1. Remove the tops from the peppers and slice each one in half lengthwise. Use a small knife to remove seeds and membranes.
2. In a small bowl, mix cream cheese, bacon, and pepper jack.
3. Place 3 teaspoons of the mixture into each sweet pepper and press down smooth. Place into the fryer basket.
4. Adjust the temperature to 400°F (205ºC) and set the timer for 8 minutes.
5. Serve warm.

Per Serving

calories: 176 | fat: 13g | protein: 7g | carbs: 4g | net carbs: 3g | fiber: 1g

Prosciutto-Wrapped Guacamole Rings

Prep time: 10 minutes | Cook time: 6 minutes | Makes 8 rings

2 avocados, halved, pitted, and peeled

3 tablespoons lime juice, plus more to taste

2 small plum tomatoes, diced

½ cup finely diced onions

2 small cloves garlic, smashed to a paste

3 tablespoons chopped fresh cilantro leaves

½ scant teaspoon fine sea salt

½ scant teaspoon ground cumin

2 small onions (about 1½-inches in diameter), cut into ½-inch-thick slices

8 slices prosciutto

1. Make the guacamole: Place the avocados and lime juice in a large bowl and mash with a fork until it reaches your desired consistency. Add the tomatoes, onions, garlic, cilantro, salt, and cumin and stir until well combined. Taste and add more lime juice if desired. Set aside half of the guacamole for serving. (Note: If you're making the guacamole ahead of time, place it in a large resealable plastic bag, squeeze out all the air, and seal it shut. It will keep in the refrigerator for up to 3 days when stored this way.)
2. Place a piece of parchment paper on a tray that fits in your freezer and place the onion slices on it, breaking the slices apart into 8 rings. Fill each ring with about 2 tablespoons of guacamole. Place the tray in the freezer for 2 hours.
3. Spray the air fryer basket with avocado oil. Preheat the air fryer to 400°F (205ºC).

4. Remove the rings from the freezer and wrap each in a slice of prosciutto. Place them in the air fryer basket, leaving space between them (if you're using a smaller air fryer, work in batches if necessary), and cook for 6 minutes, flipping halfway through. Use a spatula to remove the rings from the air fryer. Serve with the reserved half of the guacamole.
5. Store leftovers in an airtight container in the refrigerator for up to 4 days. Reheat in a preheated 400°F (205°C) air fryer for about 3 minutes, until heated through.

Per Serving

calories: 132 | fat: 9g | protein: 5g | carbs: 10g | net carbs: 6g | fiber: 4g

Cheesy Pork Rind Tortillas

Prep time: 10 minutes | Cook time: 5 minutes | Makes 4 tortillas

1 ounce (28 g) pork rinds

¾ cup shredded Mozzarella cheese

2 tablespoons full-fat cream cheese

1 large egg

1. Place pork rinds into food processor and pulse until finely ground.
2. Place Mozzarella into a large microwave-safe bowl. Break cream cheese into small pieces and add them to the bowl. Microwave for 30 seconds, or until both cheeses are melted and can easily be stirred together into a ball. Add ground pork rinds and egg to the cheese mixture.
3. Continue stirring until the mixture forms a ball. If it cools too much and cheese hardens, microwave for 10 more seconds.
4. Separate the dough into four small balls. Place each ball of dough between two sheets of parchment and roll into ¼-inch flat layer.
5. Place tortillas into the air fryer basket in single layer, working in batches if necessary.
6. Adjust the temperature to 400°F (205°C) and set the timer for 5 minutes.
7. Tortillas will be crispy and firm when fully cooked. Serve immediately.

Per Serving

calories: 145 | fat: 10g | protein: 11g | carbs: 1g | net carbs: 1g | fiber: 0g

Cheesy Pork and Chicken

Prep time: 5 minutes | Cook time: 5 minutes | Serves 2

1 ounce (28 g) pork rinds
4 ounces (113 g) shredded cooked chicken
½ cup shredded Monterey jack cheese
¼ cup sliced pickled jalapeños
¼ cup guacamole
¼ cup full-fat sour cream

1. Place pork rinds into 6-inch round baking pan. Cover with shredded chicken and Monterey jack cheese. Place pan into the air fryer basket.
2. Adjust the temperature to 370°F (188ºC) and set the timer for 5 minutes or until cheese is melted.
3. Top with jalapeños, guacamole, and sour cream. Serve immediately.

Per Serving

calories: 395 | fat: 27g | protein: 30g | carbs: 3g | net carbs: 2g | fiber: 1g

Pork Cheese Sticks

Prep time: 20 minutes | Cook time: 10 minutes | Makes 12 sticks

6 (1-ounce / 28-g) Mozzarella string cheese sticks
½ cup grated Parmesan cheese
½ ounce (14 g) pork rinds, finely ground
1 teaspoon dried parsley
2 large eggs

1. Place Mozzarella sticks on a cutting board and cut in half. Freeze 45 minutes or until firm. If freezing overnight, remove frozen sticks after 1 hour and place into airtight zip-top storage bag and place back in freezer for future use.
2. In a large bowl, mix Parmesan, ground pork rinds, and parsley.
3. In a medium bowl, whisk eggs.

4. Dip a frozen Mozzarella stick into beaten eggs and then into Parmesan mixture to coat. Repeat with remaining sticks. Place Mozzarella sticks into the air fryer basket.
5. Adjust the temperature to 400°F (205°C) and set the timer for 10 minutes or until golden.
6. Serve warm.

Per Serving

calories: 236 | fat: 13g | protein: 19g | carbs: 5g | net carbs: 5g | fiber: 0g

Cheesy Cauliflower Buns

Prep time: 15 minutes | Cook time: 12 minutes | Makes 8 buns

1 (12-ounce 340-g) steamer bag cauliflower, cooked according to package instructions

½ cup shredded Mozzarella cheese

¼ cup shredded mild Cheddar cheese

¼ cup blanched finely ground almond flour

1 large egg

½ teaspoon salt

1. Let cooked cauliflower cool about 10 minutes. Use a kitchen towel to wring out excess moisture, then place cauliflower in a food processor.
2. Add Mozzarella, Cheddar, flour, egg, and salt to the food processor and pulse twenty times until mixture is combined. It will resemble a soft, wet dough.
3. Divide mixture into eight piles. Wet your hands with water to prevent sticking, then press each pile into a flat bun shape, about ½-inch thick.
4. Cut a sheet of parchment to fit air fryer basket. Working in batches if needed, place the formed dough onto ungreased parchment in air fryer basket. Adjust the temperature to 350°F (180°C) and set the timer for 12 minutes, turning buns halfway through cooking.
5. Let buns cool 10 minutes before serving. Serve warm.

Per Serving

calories: 75 | fat: 5g | protein: 5g | carbs: 3g | net carbs: 2g | fiber: 1g

Bacon Cauliflower Skewers

Prep time: 10 minutes | Cook time: 12 minutes | Serves 4

4 slices sugar-free bacon, cut into thirds

¼ medium yellow onion, peeled and cut into 1-inch pieces

4 ounces (113 g) (about 8) cauliflower florets

1½ tablespoons olive oil

¼ teaspoon salt

¼ teaspoon garlic powder

1. Place 1 piece bacon and 2 pieces onion on a 6-inch skewer. Add a second piece bacon, and 2 cauliflower florets, followed by another piece of bacon onto skewer. Repeat with remaining ingredients and three additional skewers to make four total skewers.
2. Drizzle skewers with olive oil, then sprinkle with salt and garlic powder. Place skewers into ungreased air fryer basket. Adjust the temperature to 375°F (190ºC) and set the timer for 12 minutes, turning the skewers halfway through cooking. When done, vegetables will be tender and bacon will be crispy. Serve warm.

Per Serving

calories: 69 | fat: 5g | protein: 5g | carbs: 2g | net carbs: 1g | fiber: 1g

Crispy Cheese Salami Roll-Ups

Prep time: 5 minutes | Cook time: 4 minutes | Makes 16 roll-ups

4 ounces (113 g) cream cheese, broken into 16 equal pieces

16 (0.5-ounce / 14-g) deli slices Genoa salami

1. Place a piece of cream cheese at the edge of a slice of salami and roll to close. Secure with a toothpick. Repeat with remaining cream cheese pieces and salami.
2. Place roll-ups in an ungreased 6-inch round nonstick baking dish and place into air fryer basket. Adjust the temperature to 350°F (180ºC) and set the timer for 4 minutes. Salami will be crispy and cream cheese will be warm when done. Let cool 5 minutes before serving.

Per Serving

calories: 269 | fat: 22g | protein: 11g | carbs: 2g | net carbs: 2g | fiber: 0g

Cheesy Zucchini Fries

Prep time: 10 minutes | Cook time: 10 minutes | Serves 8

2 medium zucchini, ends removed, quartered lengthwise, and sliced into 3-inch long fries

½ teaspoon salt

⅓ cup heavy whipping cream

½ cup blanched finely ground almond flour

¾ cup grated Parmesan cheese

1 teaspoon Italian seasoning

1. Sprinkle zucchini with salt and wrap in a kitchen towel to draw out excess moisture. Let sit 2 hours.
2. Pour cream into a medium bowl. In a separate medium bowl, whisk together flour, Parmesan, and Italian seasoning.
3. Place each zucchini fry into cream, then gently shake off excess. Press each fry into dry mixture, coating each side, then place into ungreased air fryer basket. Adjust the temperature to 400°F (205°C) and set the timer for 10 minutes, turning fries halfway through cooking. Fries will be golden and crispy when done. Place on clean parchment sheet to cool 5 minutes before serving.

Per Serving

calories: 124 | fat: 10g | protein: 5g | carbs: 4g | net carbs: 3g | fiber: 1g

Aromatic Avocado Fries

Prep time: 10 minutes | Cook time: 15 minutes | Serves 6

3 firm, barely ripe avocados, halved, peeled, and pitted

2 cups pork dust (or powdered Parmesan cheese for vegetarian;)

2 teaspoons fine sea salt

2 teaspoons ground black pepper

2 teaspoons ground cumin

1 teaspoon chili powder

1 teaspoon paprika

½ teaspoon garlic powder

½ teaspoon onion powder

2 large eggs

Salsa, for serving (optional)

Fresh chopped cilantro leaves, for garnish (optional)

1. Spray the air fryer basket with avocado oil. Preheat the air fryer to 400°F (205ºC).
2. Slice the avocados into thick-cut french fry shapes.
3. In a bowl, mix together the pork dust, salt, pepper, and seasonings.
4. In a separate shallow bowl, beat the eggs.
5. Dip the avocado fries into the beaten eggs and shake off any excess, then dip them into the pork dust mixture. Use your hands to press the breading into each fry.
6. Spray the fries with avocado oil and place them in the air fryer basket in a single layer, leaving space between them. If there are too many fries to fit in a single layer, work in batches. Cook in the air fryer for 13 to 15 minutes, until golden brown, flipping after 5 minutes.
7. Serve with salsa, if desired, and garnish with fresh chopped cilantro, if desired. Best served fresh.
8. Store leftovers in an airtight container in the fridge for up to 5 days. Reheat in a preheated 400°F (205ºC) air fryer for 3 minutes, or until heated through.

Per Serving

calories: 282 | fat: 22g | protein: 15g | carbs: 9g | net carbs: 2g | fiber: 7g

Cheesy Pickle Spear

Prep time: 40 minutes | Cook time: 10 minutes | Serves 4

4 dill pickle spears, halved lengthwise

¼ cup ranch dressing

½ cup blanched finely ground almond flour

½ cup grated Parmesan cheese

2 tablespoons dry ranch seasoning

1. Wrap spears in a kitchen towel 30 minutes to soak up excess pickle juice.

2. Pour ranch dressing into a medium bowl and add pickle spears. In a separate medium bowl, mix flour, Parmesan, and ranch seasoning.
3. Remove each spear from ranch dressing and shake off excess. Press gently into dry mixture to coat all sides. Place spears into ungreased air fryer basket. Adjust the temperature to 400°F (205ºC) and set the timer for 10 minutes, turning spears three times during cooking. Serve warm.

Per Serving

calories: 160 | fat: 11g | protein: 7g | carbs: 8g | net carbs: 6g | fiber: 2g

Crispy Pepperoni Chips

Prep time: 5 minutes | Cook time: 8 minutes | Serves 2

14 slices pepperoni

1. Place pepperoni slices into ungreased air fryer basket. Adjust the temperature to 350°F (180ºC) and set the timer for 8 minutes. Pepperoni will be browned and crispy when done. Let cool 5 minutes before serving. Store in airtight container at room temperature up to 3 days.

Per Serving

calories: 69 | fat: 5g | protein: 3g | carbs: 0g | net carbs: 0g | fiber: 0g

Vinegary Pork Belly Chips

Prep time: 5 minutes | Cook time: 12 minutes | Serves 4

1 pound (454 g) slab pork belly

½ cup apple cider vinegar

Fine sea salt

FOR SERVING (OPTIONAL):

Guacamole

Pico de gallo

1. Slice the pork belly into ⅛-inch-thick strips and place them in a shallow dish. Pour in the vinegar and stir to coat the pork belly. Place in the fridge to marinate for 30 minutes.

2. Spray the air fryer basket with avocado oil. Preheat the air fryer to 400°F (205ºC).
3. Remove the pork belly from the vinegar and place the strips in the air fryer basket in a single layer, leaving space between them. Cook in the air fryer for 10 to 12 minutes, until crispy, flipping after 5 minutes. Remove from the air fryer and sprinkle with salt. Serve with guacamole and pico de gallo, if desired.
4. Best served fresh. Store leftovers in an airtight container in the fridge for up to 5 days. Reheat in a preheated 400°F (205ºC) air fryer for 5 minutes, or until heated through, flipping halfway through.

Per Serving

calories: 240 | fat: 21g | protein: 13g | carbs: 0g | net carbs: 0g | fiber: 0g

Air Fried Kale Chips

Prep time: 5 minutes | Cook time: 10 minutes | Makes 8 cups

½ teaspoon dried chives
½ teaspoon dried dill weed
½ teaspoon dried parsley
¼ teaspoon garlic powder
¼ teaspoon onion powder
⅛ teaspoon fine sea salt
⅛ teaspoon ground black pepper
2 large bunches kale

1. Spray the air fryer basket with avocado oil. Preheat the air fryer to 360°F (182ºC).
2. Place the seasonings, salt, and pepper in a small bowl and mix well.
3. Wash the kale and pat completely dry. Use a sharp knife to carve out the thick inner stems, then spray the leaves with avocado oil and sprinkle them with the seasoning mix.
4. Place the kale leaves in the air fryer in a single layer and cook for 10 minutes, shaking and rotating the chips halfway through. Transfer the baked chips to a baking sheet to cool completely and crisp up. Repeat with the remaining kale. Sprinkle the cooled chips with salt before serving, if desired.
5. Kale chips can be stored in an airtight container at room temperature for up to 1 week, but they are best eaten within 3 days.

Per Serving

calories: 11 | fat: 1g | protein: 1g | carbs: 2g | net carbs: 1g | fiber: 1g

Prosciutto Pierogi

Prep time: 15 minutes | Cook time: 20 minutes | Makes 4 pierogi

1 cup chopped cauliflower

2 tablespoons diced onions

1 tablespoon unsalted butter (or lard or bacon fat for dairy-free), melted

pinch of fine sea salt

½ cup shredded sharp Cheddar cheese (about 2 ounces / 57 g) (or Kite Hill brand cream cheese style spread, softened, for dairy-free)

8 slices prosciutto

Fresh oregano leaves, for garnish (optional)

1. Preheat the air fryer to 350°F (180°C). Lightly grease a 7-inch pie pan or a casserole dish that will fit in your air fryer.
2. Make the filling: Place the cauliflower and onion in the pan. Drizzle with the melted butter and sprinkle with the salt. Using your hands, mix everything together, making sure the cauliflower is coated in the butter.
3. Place the cauliflower mixture in the air fryer and cook for 10 minutes, until fork-tender, stirring halfway through.
4. Transfer the cauliflower mixture to a food processor or high-powered blender. Spray the air fryer basket with avocado oil and increase the air fryer temperature to 400°F (205°C).
5. Pulse the cauliflower mixture in the food processor until smooth. Stir in the cheese.
6. Assemble the pierogi: Lay 1 slice of prosciutto on a sheet of parchment paper with a short end toward you. Lay another slice of prosciutto on top of it at a right angle, forming a cross. Spoon about 2 heaping tablespoons of the filling into the center of the cross.
7. Fold each arm of the prosciutto cross over the filling to form a square, making sure that the filling is well covered. Using your fingers, press down around the filling to even out the square shape. Repeat with the rest of the prosciutto and filling.
8. Spray the pierogi with avocado oil and place them in the air fryer basket. Cook for 10 minutes, or until crispy.
9. Garnish with oregano before serving, if desired. Store leftovers in an airtight container in the fridge for up to 4 days. Reheat in a preheated 400°F (205°C) air fryer for 3 minutes, or until heated through.

Per Serving

calories: 150 | fat: 11g | protein: 11g | carbs: 2g | net carbs: 1g | fiber: 1g

Air Fried Brussels Sprout

Prep time: 20 minutes | Cook time: 15 minutes | Serves 4

1 pound (454 g) Brussels sprouts, ends and yellow leaves removed and halved lengthwise

Salt and black pepper, to taste

1 tablespoon toasted sesame oil

1 teaspoon fennel seeds

Chopped fresh parsley, for garnish

1. Place the Brussels sprouts, salt, pepper, sesame oil, and fennel seeds in a resealable plastic bag. Seal the bag and shake to coat.
2. Air-fry at 380 degrees F (193ºC) for 15 minutes or until tender. Make sure to flip them over halfway through the cooking time.
3. Serve sprinkled with fresh parsley. Bon appétit!

Per Serving

calories: 174 | fat: 3g | protein: 3g | carbs: 9g | net carbs: 5g | fiber: 4g

Savory Eggplant

Prep time: 45 minutes | Cook time: 13 minutes | Serves 4

1 eggplant, peeled and thinly sliced

Salt, to taste

½ cup almond meal

¼ cup olive oil

½ cup water

1 teaspoon garlic powder

½ teaspoon dried dill weed

½ teaspoon ground black pepper, to taste

1. Salt the eggplant slices and let them stay for about 30 minutes. Squeeze the eggplant slices and rinse them under cold running water.
2. Toss the eggplant slices with the other ingredients. Cook at 390 degrees F (199ºC) for 13 minutes, working in batches.

3. Serve with a sauce for dipping. Bon appétit!

Per Serving

calories: 241 | fat: 21g | protein: 4g | carbs: 9g | net carbs: 4g | fiber: 5g

Golden Cheese Crisps

Prep time: 10 minutes | Cook time: 12 minutes | Serves 2

½ cup shredded Cheddar cheese

1 egg white

1. Preheat the air fryer to 400°F (205ºC). Place a piece of parchment paper in the bottom of the air fryer basket.
2. In a medium bowl, combine the cheese and egg white, stirring with a fork until thoroughly combined.
3. Place small scoops of the cheese mixture in a single layer in the basket of the air fryer (about 1-inch apart). Use the fork to spread the mixture as thin as possible. Air fry for 10 to 12 minutes until the crisps are golden brown. Let cool for a few minutes before transferring them to a plate. Store at room temperature in an airtight container for up to 3 days.

Per Serving

calories: 120 | fat: 10g | protein: 9g | carbs: 1g | net carbs: 1g | fiber: 0g

Broccoli Fries with Spicy Dip

Prep time: 15 minutes | Cook time: 6 minutes | Serves 4

¾ pound (340g) broccoli florets

½ teaspoon onion powder

1 teaspoon granulated garlic

½ teaspoon cayenne pepper

Sea salt and ground black pepper, to taste

2 tablespoons sesame oil

4 tablespoons Parmesan cheese, preferably freshly grated

Spicy Dip:

¼ cup mayonnaise

¼ cup Greek yogurt

¼ teaspoon Dijon mustard

1 teaspoon keto hot sauce

1. Start by preheating the Air Fryer to 400 degrees F (205ºC).
2. Blanch the broccoli in salted boiling water until al dente, about 3 to 4 minutes. Drain well and transfer to the lightly greased Air Fryer basket.
3. Add the onion powder, garlic, cayenne pepper, salt, black pepper, sesame oil, and Parmesan cheese.
4. Cook for 6 minutes, tossing halfway through the cooking time.
5. Meanwhile, mix all of the spicy dip ingredients. Serve broccoli fries with chilled dipping sauce. Bon appétit!

Per Serving

calories: 219 | fat: 19g | protein: 5g | carbs: 9g | net carbs: 6g | fiber: 3g

Cheesy Broccoli

Prep time: 20 minutes | Cook time: 20 minutes | Serves 6

2 eggs, well whisked

2 cups Colby cheese, shredded

½ cup almond meal

2 tablespoons sesame seeds

Seasoned salt, to taste

¼ teaspoon ground black pepper, or more to taste

1 head broccoli, grated

1 cup Parmesan cheese, grated

1. Thoroughly combine the eggs, Colby cheese, almond meal, sesame seeds, salt, black pepper, and broccoli to make the consistency of dough.
2. Chill for 1 hour and shape into small balls; roll the patties over Parmesan cheese. Spritz them with cooking oil on all sides.
3. Cook at 360 degrees F (182ºC) for 10 minutes. Check for doneness and return to the Air Fryer for 8 to 10 more minutes. Serve with a sauce for dipping. Bon appétit!

Per Serving

calories: 322 | fat: 23g | protein: 19g | carbs: 9g | net carbs: 6g | fiber: 3g

Spinach Melts with Chilled Sauce

Prep time: 20 minutes | Cook time: 14 minutes | Serves 4

Spinach Melts:

2 cups spinach, torn into pieces

1 ½ cups cauliflower

1 tablespoon sesame oil

½ cup scallions, chopped

2 garlic cloves, minced

½ cup almond flour

¼ cup coconut flour

1 teaspoon baking powder

½ teaspoon sea salt

½ teaspoon ground black pepper

¼ teaspoon dried dill

½ teaspoon dried basil

1 cup Cheddar cheese, shredded

Parsley Yogurt Dip:

½ cup Greek-Style yoghurt

2 tablespoons mayonnaise

2 tablespoons fresh parsley, chopped

1 tablespoon fresh lemon juice

½ teaspoon garlic, smashed

1. Place spinach in a mixing dish; pour in hot water. Drain and rinse well.
2. Add cauliflower to the steamer basket; steam until the cauliflower is tender about 5 minutes.
3. Mash the cauliflower; add the remaining ingredients for Spinach Melts and mix to combine well. Shape the mixture into patties and transfer them to the lightly greased cooking basket.
4. Bake at 330 degrees F (166ºC) for 14 minutes or until thoroughly heated.

5. Meanwhile, make your dipping sauce by whisking the remaining ingredients. Place in your refrigerator until ready to serve.
6. Serve the Spinach Melts with the chilled sauce on the side. Enjoy!

Per Serving

calories: 301 | fat: 25g | protein: 11g | carbs: 9g | net carbs: 5g | fiber: 4g

Aromatic Bacon Shrimp

Prep time: 45 minutes | Cook time: 8 minutes | Serves 10

1¼ pounds (567g) shrimp, peeled and deveined

1 teaspoon paprika

½ teaspoon ground black pepper

½ teaspoon red pepper flakes, crushed

1 tablespoon salt

1 teaspoon chili powder

1 tablespoon shallot powder

¼ teaspoon cumin powder

1¼ pounds (567g) thin bacon slices

1. Toss the shrimps with all the seasoning until they are coated well.
2. Next, wrap a slice of bacon around the shrimps, securing with a toothpick; repeat with the remaining ingredients; chill for 30 minutes.
3. Air-fry them at 360 degrees F (182ºC) for 7 to 8 minutes, working in batches. Serve with cocktail sticks if desired. Enjoy!

Per Serving

calories: 282 | fat: 22g | protein: 19g | carbs: 2g | net carbs: 1g | fiber: 1g

Roasted Zucchini

Prep time: 20 minutes | Cook time: 18 minutes | Serves 6

1½ pounds (680g) zucchini, peeled and cut into ½-inch chunks

2 tablespoons melted coconut oil

A pinch of coarse salt

A pinch of pepper

2 tablespoons sage, finely chopped

Zest of 1 small-sized lemon

⅛ teaspoon ground allspice

1. Toss the squash chunks with the other items.
2. Roast in the Air Fryer cooking basket at 350 degrees F (180ºC) for 10 minutes.
3. Pause the machine, and turn the temperature to 400 degrees F; stir and roast for additional 8 minutes. Bon appétit!

Per Serving

calories: 270 | fat: 15g | protein: 3g | carbs: 5g | net carbs: 4g | fiber: 1g

Cheesy Meatball

Prep time: 20 minutes | Cook time: 18 minutes | Serves 8

½ teaspoon fine sea salt

1 cup Romano cheese, grated

3 cloves garlic, minced

1½ pound (680g) ground pork

½ cup scallions, finely chopped

2 eggs, well whisked

⅓ teaspoon cumin powder

⅔ teaspoon ground black pepper, or more to taste

2 teaspoons basil

1. Simply combine all the ingredients in a large-sized mixing bowl.
2. Shape into bite-sized balls; cook the meatballs in the air fryer for 18 minutes at 345 degrees F (174ºC). Serve with some tangy sauce such as marinara sauce if desired. Bon appétit!

Per Serving

calories: 350 | fat: 25g | protein: 28g | carbs: 2g | net carbs: 1g | fiber: 1g

Pork Meatball

Prep time: 25 minutes | Cook time: 17 minutes | Serves 8

1 teaspoon cayenne pepper

2 teaspoons mustard

2 tablespoons Brie cheese, grated

5 garlic cloves, minced

2 small-sized yellow onions, peeled and chopped

1½ pounds (680g) ground pork

Sea salt and freshly ground black pepper, to taste

1. Mix all of the above ingredients until everything is well incorporated.
2. Now, form the mixture into balls (the size of golf a ball).
3. Cook for 17 minutes at 375 degrees F (190ºC). Serve with your favorite sauce.

Per Serving

calories: 275 | fat: 18g | protein: 3g | carbs: 3g | net carbs: 2g | fiber: 1g

Beef Cheese Burger

Prep time: 20 minutes | Cook time: 15 minutes | Serves 4

1 tablespoon Dijon mustard

2 tablespoons minced scallions

1 pound (454 g) ground beef

1½ teaspoons minced green garlic

½ teaspoon cumin

Salt and ground black pepper, to taste

12 cherry tomatoes

12 cubes Cheddar cheese

1. In a large-sized mixing dish, place the mustard, ground beef, cumin, scallions, garlic, salt, and pepper; mix with your hands or a spatula so that everything is evenly coated.

2. Form into 12 meatballs and cook them in the preheated Air Fryer for 15 minutes at 375 degrees F (190ºC). Air-fry until they are cooked in the middle.
3. Thread cherry tomatoes, mini burgers and cheese on cocktail sticks. Bon appétit!

Per Serving

calories: 469 | fat: 30g | protein: 3g | carbs: 4g | net carbs: 3g | fiber: 1g

Cheesy Chicken Nuggets

Prep time: 20 minutes | Cook time: 12 minutes | Serves 6

1 pound (454 g) chicken breasts, slice into tenders
½ teaspoon cayenne pepper
Salt and black pepper, to taste
¼ cup almond meal
1 egg, whisked
½ cup Parmesan cheese, freshly grated
¼ cup mayo
¼ cup no-sugar-added barbecue sauce

1. Pat the chicken tenders dry with a kitchen towel. Season with the cayenne pepper, salt, and black pepper.
2. Dip the chicken tenders into the almond meal, followed by the egg. Press the chicken tenders into the Parmesan cheese, coating evenly.
3. Place the chicken tenders in the lightly greased Air Fryer basket. Cook at 360 degrees for 9 to 12 minutes, turning them over to cook evenly.
4. In a mixing bowl, thoroughly combine the mayonnaise with the barbecue sauce. Serve the chicken nuggets with the sauce for dipping. Bon appétit!

Per Serving

calories: 268 | fat: 18g | protein: 2g | carbs: 4g | net carbs: 3g | fiber: 1g

Crisp Cauliflower

Prep time: 20 minutes | Cook time: 12 minutes | Serves 2

3 cups cauliflower florets

2 tablespoons sesame oil

1 teaspoon onion powder

1 teaspoon garlic powder

1 teaspoon thyme

1 teaspoon sage

1 teaspoon rosemary

Sea salt and cracked black pepper, to taste

1 teaspoon paprika

1. Start by preheating your Air Fryer to 400 degrees F (205ºC).
2. Toss the cauliflower with the remaining ingredients; toss to coat well.
3. Cook for 12 minutes, shaking the cooking basket halfway through the cooking time. They will crisp up as they cool. Bon appétit!

Per Serving

calories: 160 | fat: 14g | protein: 3g | carbs: 8g | net carbs: 5g | fiber: 3g

Roast Chicken with Teriyaki Sauce

Prep time: 40 minutes | Cook time: 26 minutes | Serves 6

1½ pounds (680g) chicken drumettes

Sea salt and cracked black pepper, to taste

2 tablespoons fresh chives, roughly chopped

Teriyaki Sauce:

1 tablespoon sesame oil

¼ cup coconut aminos

½ cup water

½ teaspoon Five-spice powder

2 tablespoons rice wine vinegar

½ teaspoon fresh ginger, grated

2 cloves garlic, crushed

1. Start by preheating your Air Fryer to 380 degrees F (193ºC). Rub the chicken drumettes with salt and cracked black pepper.
2. Cook in the preheated Air Fryer approximately 15 minutes. Turn them over and cook an additional 7 minutes.
3. While the chicken drumettes are roasting, combine the sesame oil, coconut aminos, water, Five-spice powder, vinegar, ginger, and garlic in a pan over medium heat. Cook for 5 minutes, stirring occasionally.
4. Now, reduce the heat and let it simmer until the glaze thickens.
5. After that, brush the glaze all over the chicken drumettes. Air-fry for a further 6 minutes or until the surface is crispy. Serve topped with the remaining glaze and garnished with fresh chives. Bon appétit!

Per Serving

calories: 301 | fat: 21g | protein: 22g | carbs: 4g | net carbs: 3g | fiber: 1g

Zucchini and Bacon Cheese Cake

Prep time: 22 minutes | Cook time: 13 minutes | Serves 4

1/3 cup Swiss cheese, grated

1/3 teaspoon fine sea salt

1/3 teaspoon baking powder

1/3 cup scallions, finely chopped

½ tablespoon fresh basil, finely chopped

1 zucchini, trimmed and grated

½ teaspoon freshly cracked black pepper

1 teaspoon Mexican oregano

1 cup bacon, chopped

¼ cup almond meal

¼ cup coconut flour

2 small eggs, lightly beaten

1 cup Cotija cheese, grated

1. Mix all ingredients, except for Cotija cheese, until everything is well combined.
2. Then, gently flatten each ball. Spritz the cakes with a nonstick cooking oil.
3. Bake your cakes for 13 minutes at 305 degrees F (152ºC); work with batches. Serve warm with tomato ketchup and mayonnaise.

Per Serving

calories: 311 | fat: 25g | protein: 18g | carbs: 5g | net carbs: 3g | fiber: 2g

Cheesy Tomato Chips

Prep time: 15 minutes | Cook time: 10 minutes | Serves 4

4 Roma tomatoes, sliced

2 tablespoons olive oil

Sea salt and white pepper, to taste

1 teaspoon Italian seasoning mix

½ cup Parmesan cheese, grated

1. Start by preheating your Air Fryer to 350 degrees F (180ºC). Generously grease the Air Fryer basket with nonstick cooking oil.
2. Toss the sliced tomatoes with the remaining ingredients. Transfer them to the cooking basket without overlapping.
3. Cook in the preheated Air Fryer for 5 minutes. Shake the cooking basket and cook an additional 5 minutes. Work in batches.
4. Serve with Mediterranean aioli for dipping, if desired. Bon appétit!

Per Serving

calories: 130 | fat: 10g | protein: 5g | carbs: 6g | net carbs: 5g | fiber: 1g

Air Fried Bell Pepper

Prep time: 20 minutes | Cook time: 7 minutes | Serves 4

1 egg, beaten

½ cup Parmesan, grated

1 teaspoon sea salt

½ teaspoon red pepper flakes, crushed

¾ pound (340g) bell peppers, seeded and cut to ¼-inch strips

2 tablespoons olive oil

1. In a mixing bowl, combine together the egg, Parmesan, salt, and red pepper flakes; mix to combine well.
2. Dip bell peppers into the batter and transfer them to the cooking basket. Brush with the olive oil.
3. Cook in the preheated Air Fryer at 390 degrees F (199ºC) for 4 minutes. Shake the basket and cook for a further 3 minutes. Work in batches.
4. Taste, adjust the seasonings and serve. Bon appétit!

Per Serving

calories: 163 | fat: 11g | protein: 6g | carbs: 10g | net carbs: 9g | fiber: 1g

Baked Spinach Chips

Prep time: 20 minutes | Cook time: 10 minutes | Serves 3

3 cups fresh spinach leaves
1 tablespoon extra-virgin olive oil
1 teaspoon sea salt
½ teaspoon cayenne pepper
1 teaspoon garlic powder
Chili Yogurt Dip:
¼ cup yogurt
2 tablespoons mayonnaise
½ teaspoon chili powder

1. Toss the spinach leaves with the olive oil and seasonings.
2. Bake in the preheated Air Fryer at 350 degrees F (180ºC) for 10 minutes, shaking the cooking basket occasionally.
3. Bake until the edges brown, working in batches.
4. In the meantime, make the sauce by whisking all ingredients in a mixing dish. Serve immediately.

Per Serving
calories: 128 | fat: 12g | protein: 2g | carbs: 3g | net carbs: 2g | fiber: 1g

Scallops and Bacon Kabobs

Prep time: 40 minutes | Cook time: 6 minutes | Serves 6

1 pound (454 g) sea scallops
½ cup coconut milk
1 tablespoon vermouth
Sea salt and ground black pepper, to taste
½ pound (227g) bacon, diced
1 shallot, diced
1 teaspoon garlic powder
1 teaspoon paprika

1. In a ceramic bowl, place the sea scallops, coconut milk, vermouth, salt, and black pepper; let it marinate for 30 minutes.
2. Assemble the skewers alternating the scallops, bacon, and shallots. Sprinkle garlic powder and paprika all over the skewers.
3. Bake in the preheated air Fryer at 400 degrees F (205ºC) for 6 minutes. Serve warm and enjoy!

Per Serving

calories: 228 | fat: 15g | protein: 15g | carbs: 5g | net carbs: 5g | fiber: 0g

Bacon and Egg Bites

Prep time: 20 minutes | Cook time: 13 minutes | Serves 4

6 ounces (170 g) (about 9 slices) reduced-sodium bacon

2 hard-boiled eggs, chopped

Flesh of ½ avocado, chopped

2 tablespoons unsalted butter, softened

2 tablespoons mayonnaise

1 jalapeño pepper, seeded and finely chopped

2 tablespoons chopped fresh cilantro

Juice of ½ lime

Salt and freshly ground black pepper

1. Arrange the bacon in a single layer in the air fryer basket (it's OK if the bacon sits a bit on the sides). Set the air fryer to 350°F (180ºC) and cook for 10 minutes. Check for crispiness and cook for 2 to 3 minutes longer if needed. Transfer the bacon to a paper towel–lined plate and let cool completely. Reserve 2 tablespoons of bacon grease from the bottom of the air fryer basket. Finely chop the bacon and set aside in a small, shallow bowl.
2. In a large bowl, combine the eggs, avocado, butter, mayonnaise, jalapeño, cilantro, and lime juice. Mash into a smooth paste with a fork or potato smasher. Season to taste with salt and pepper.
3. Add the reserved bacon grease to the egg mixture and stir gently until thoroughly combined. Cover and refrigerate for 30 minutes, or until the mixture is firm.
4. Divide the mixture into 12 equal portions and shape into balls. Roll the balls in the chopped bacon bits until completely coated.

Per Serving

calories: 330 | fat: 31g | protein: 10g | carbs: 2g | net carbs: 2g | fiber: 0g

Side Dishes

Kohlrabi Fries

Prep time: 10 minutes | Cook time: 30 minutes | Serves 4

2 pounds (907 g) kohlrabi, peeled and cut into ¼–½-inch fries

2 tablespoons olive oil

Salt and freshly ground black pepper

1. Preheat the air fryer to 400°F (205°C).
2. In a large bowl, combine the kohlrabi and olive oil. Season to taste with salt and black pepper. Toss gently until thoroughly coated.
3. Working in batches if necessary, spread the kohlrabi in a single layer in the air fryer basket. Pausing halfway through the cooking time to shake the basket, air fry for 20 to 30 minutes until the fries are lightly browned and crunchy.

Per Serving

calories: 120 | fat: 7g | protein: 4g | carbs: 14g | net carbs: 12g | fiber: 2g

Air Fried Bok Choy

Prep time: 10 minutes | Cook time: 10 minutes | Serves 4

2 tablespoons olive oil

2 tablespoons coconut aminos

2 teaspoons sesame oil

2 teaspoons chili-garlic sauce

2 cloves garlic, minced

1 head (about 1 pound / 454 g) bok choy, sliced lengthwise into quarters

2 teaspoons black sesame seeds

1. Preheat the air fryer to 400°F (205°C).
2. In a large bowl, combine the olive oil, coconut aminos, sesame oil, chili-garlic sauce, and garlic. Add the bok choy and toss, massaging the leaves with your hands if necessary, until thoroughly coated.
3. Arrange the bok choy in the basket of the air fryer. Pausing about halfway through the cooking time to shake the basket, air fry for 7 to 10 minutes until the bok choy is tender

and the tips of the leaves begin to crisp. Remove from the basket and let cool for a few minutes before coarsely chopping. Serve sprinkled with the sesame seeds.

Per Serving

calories: 100 | fat: 8g | protein: 2g | carbs: 4g | net carbs: 3g | fiber: 1g

Brussels Sprouts with Pecan

Prep time: 10 minutes | Cook time: 30 minutes | Serves 4

½ cup pecans

1½ pounds (680g) fresh Brussels sprouts, trimmed and quartered

2 tablespoons olive oil

Salt and freshly ground black pepper

¼ cup crumbled Gorgonzola cheese

1. Spread the pecans in a single layer of the air fryer and set the heat to 350°F (180°C). Air fry for 3 to 5 minutes until the pecans are lightly browned and fragrant. Transfer the pecans to a plate and continue preheating the air fryer, increasing the heat to 400°F (205°C).
2. In a large bowl, toss the Brussels sprouts with the olive oil and season with salt and black pepper to taste.
3. Working in batches if necessary, arrange the Brussels sprouts in a single layer in the air fryer basket. Pausing halfway through the baking time to shake the basket, air fry for 20 to 25 minutes until the sprouts are tender and starting to brown on the edges.
4. Transfer the sprouts to a serving bowl and top with the toasted pecans and Gorgonzola. Serve warm or at room temperature.

Per Serving

calories: 250 | fat: 19g | protein: 9g | carbs: 17g | net carbs: 9g | fiber: 8g

Brussels Sprouts with Bacon

Prep time: 5 minutes | Cook time: 12 minutes | Serves 4

2 cups trimmed and halved fresh Brussels sprouts

2 tablespoons olive oil

¼ teaspoon salt

¼ teaspoon ground black pepper

2 tablespoons balsamic vinegar

2 slices cooked sugar-free bacon, crumbled

1. In a large bowl, toss Brussels sprouts in olive oil, then sprinkle with salt and pepper. Place into ungreased air fryer basket. Adjust the temperature to 375°F (190ºC) and set the timer for 12 minutes, shaking the basket halfway through cooking. Brussels sprouts will be tender and browned when done.
2. Place sprouts in a large serving dish and drizzle with balsamic vinegar. Sprinkle bacon over top. Serve warm.

Per Serving

calories: 112 | fat: 9g | protein: 3g | carbs: 5g | net carbs: 3g | fiber: 2g

Bacon-Wrapped Asparagus

Prep time: 5 minutes | Cook time: 10 minutes | Serves 4

8 slices reduced-sodium bacon, cut in half

16 thick (about 1 pound / 454 g) asparagus spears, trimmed of woody ends

1. Preheat the air fryer to 350°F (180ºC).
2. Wrap a half piece of bacon around the center of each stalk of asparagus.
3. Working in batches, if necessary, arrange seam-side down in a single layer in the air fryer basket. Cook for 10 minutes until the bacon is crisp and the stalks are tender.

Per Serving

calories: 110 | fat: 7g | protein: 8g | carbs: 5g | net carbs: 3g | fiber: 2g

Air Fried Asparagus

Prep time: 5 minutes | Cook time: 12 minutes | Serves 4

1 tablespoon olive oil

1 pound (454 g) asparagus spears, ends trimmed

¼ teaspoon salt

¼ teaspoon ground black pepper

1 tablespoon salted butter, melted

1. In a large bowl, drizzle olive oil over asparagus spears and sprinkle with salt and pepper.
2. Place spears into ungreased air fryer basket. Adjust the temperature to 375°F (190ºC) and set the timer for 12 minutes, shaking the basket halfway through cooking. Asparagus will be lightly browned and tender when done.
3. Transfer to a large dish and drizzle with butter. Serve warm.

Per Serving

calories: 73 | fat: 6g | protein: 2g | carbs: 4g | net carbs: 2g | fiber: 2g

Cheesy Asparagus

Prep time: 10 minutes | Cook time: 18 minutes | Serves 4

½ cup heavy whipping cream

½ cup grated Parmesan cheese

2 ounces (57 g) cream cheese, softened

1 pound (454 g) asparagus, ends trimmed, chopped into 1-inch pieces

¼ teaspoon salt

¼ teaspoon ground black pepper

1. In a medium bowl, whisk together heavy cream, Parmesan, and cream cheese until combined.
2. Place asparagus into an ungreased 6-inch round nonstick baking dish. Pour cheese mixture over top and sprinkle with salt and pepper.
3. Place dish into air fryer basket. Adjust the temperature to 350°F (180ºC) and set the timer for 18 minutes. Asparagus will be tender when done. Serve warm.

Per Serving

calories: 221 | fat: 18g | protein: 7g | carbs: 7g | net carbs: 5g | fiber: 2g

Cheesy Bean Mushroon Casserole

Prep time: 10 minutes | Cook time: 12 minutes | Serves 4

1 pound (454 g) fresh green beans, ends trimmed, strings removed, and chopped into 2-inch pieces

1 (8-ounce / 227-g) package sliced brown mushrooms

½ onion, sliced

1 clove garlic, minced

1 tablespoon olive oil

½ teaspoon salt

¼ teaspoon freshly ground black pepper

4 ounces (113 g) cream cheese

½ cup chicken stock

¼ teaspoon ground nutmeg

½ cup grated Cheddar cheese

1. Preheat the air fryer to 400°F (205ºC). Coat a 6-cup casserole dish with olive oil and set aside.
2. In a large bowl, combine the green beans, mushrooms, onion, garlic, olive oil, salt, and pepper. Toss until the vegetables are thoroughly coated with the oil and seasonings.
3. Transfer the mixture to the air fryer basket. Pausing halfway through the cooking time to shake the basket, air fry for 10 minutes until tender.
4. While the vegetables are cooking, in a 2-cup glass measuring cup, warm the cream cheese and chicken stock in the microwave on high for 1 to 2 minutes until the cream cheese is melted. Add the nutmeg and whisk until smooth.
5. Transfer the vegetables to the prepared casserole dish and pour the cream cheese mixture over the top. Top with the Cheddar cheese. Air fry for another 10 minutes until the cheese is melted and beginning to brown.

Per Serving

calories: 250 | fat: 19g | protein: 10g | carbs: 14g | net carbs: 10g | fiber: 4g

Crispy Green Beans

Prep time: 5 minutes | Cook time: 8 minutes | Serves 4

2 teaspoons olive oil

½ pound (227g) fresh green beans, ends trimmed

¼ teaspoon salt

¼ teaspoon ground black pepper

1. In a large bowl, drizzle olive oil over green beans and sprinkle with salt and pepper.
2. Place green beans into ungreased air fryer basket. Adjust the temperature to 350°F (180ºC) and set the timer for 8 minutes, shaking the basket two times during cooking. Green beans will be dark golden and crispy at the edges when done. Serve warm.

Per Serving

calories: 37 | fat: 2g | protein: 1g | carbs: 4g | net carbs: 2g | fiber: 2g

Air Fried Zucchini Salad

Prep time: 5 minutes | Cook time: 7 minutes | Serves 4

2 medium zucchini, thinly sliced
5 tablespoons olive oil, divided
¼ cup chopped fresh parsley
2 tablespoons chopped fresh mint
Zest and juice of ½ lemon
1 clove garlic, minced
¼ cup crumbled feta cheese
Freshly ground black pepper

1. Preheat the air fryer to 400°F (205ºC).
2. In a large bowl, toss the zucchini slices with 1 tablespoon of the olive oil.
3. Working in batches if necessary, arrange the zucchini slices in an even layer in the air fryer basket. Pausing halfway through the cooking time to shake the basket, air fry for 5 to 7 minutes until soft and lightly browned on each side.
4. Meanwhile, in a small bowl, combine the remaining 4 tablespoons olive oil, parsley, mint, lemon zest, lemon juice, and garlic.
5. Arrange the zucchini on a plate and drizzle with the dressing. Sprinkle the feta and black pepper on top. Serve warm or at room temperature.

Per Serving

calories: 195 | fat: 19g | protein: 3g | carbs: 5g | net carbs: 4g | fiber: 1g

Zucchini Fritters

Prep time: 15 minutes | Cook time: 10 minutes | Serves 4

2 zucchini, grated (about 1 pound / 454 g)

1 teaspoon salt

¼ cup almond flour

¼ cup grated Parmesan cheese

1 large egg

¼ teaspoon dried thyme

¼ teaspoon ground turmeric

¼ teaspoon freshly ground black pepper

1 tablespoon olive oil

½ lemon, sliced into wedges

1. Preheat the air fryer to 400°F (205°C). Cut a piece of parchment paper to fit slightly smaller than the bottom of the air fryer.
2. Place the zucchini in a large colander and sprinkle with the salt. Let sit for 5 to 10 minutes. Squeeze as much liquid as you can from the zucchini and place in a large mixing bowl. Add the almond flour, Parmesan, egg, thyme, turmeric, and black pepper. Stir gently until thoroughly combined.
3. Shape the mixture into 8 patties and arrange on the parchment paper. Brush lightly with the olive oil. Pausing halfway through the cooking time to turn the patties, air fry for 10 minutes until golden brown. Serve warm with the lemon wedges.

Per Serving

calories: 190 | fat: 16g | protein: 6g | carbs: 8g | net carbs: 6g | fiber: 2g

Zucchini and Tomato Boats

Prep time: 5 minutes | Cook time: 10 minutes | Serves 4

1 large zucchini, ends removed, halved lengthwise

6 grape tomatoes, quartered

¼ teaspoon salt

¼ cup feta cheese

1 tablespoon balsamic vinegar

1 tablespoon olive oil

1. Use a spoon to scoop out 2 tablespoons from center of each zucchini half, making just enough space to fill with tomatoes and feta.
2. Place tomatoes evenly in centers of zucchini halves and sprinkle with salt. Place into ungreased air fryer basket. Adjust the temperature to 350°F (180ºC) and set the timer for 10 minutes. When done, zucchini will be tender.
3. Transfer boats to a serving tray and sprinkle with feta, then drizzle with vinegar and olive oil. Serve warm.

Per Serving

calories: 74 | fat: 5g | protein: 2g | carbs: 4g | net carbs: 3g | fiber: 1g

Air Fried Cauliflower

Prep time: 15 minutes | Cook time: 20 minutes | Serves 4

¼ cup olive oil

2 teaspoons curry powder

½ teaspoon salt

¼ teaspoon freshly ground black pepper

1 head cauliflower, cut into bite-size florets

½ red onion, sliced

2 tablespoons freshly chopped parsley, for garnish (optional)

1. Preheat the air fryer to 400°F (205ºC).
2. In a large bowl, combine the olive oil, curry powder, salt, and pepper. Add the cauliflower and onion. Toss gently until the vegetables are completely coated with the oil mixture. Transfer the vegetables to the basket of the air fryer.
3. Pausing about halfway through the cooking time to shake the basket, air fry for 20 minutes until the cauliflower is tender and beginning to brown. Top with the parsley, if desired, before serving.

Per Serving

calories: 165 | fat: 14g | protein: 3g | carbs: 10g | net carbs: 6g | fiber: 4g

Cheesy Cauliflower Tots

Prep time: 15 minutes | Cook time: 12 minutes | Serves 16 tots

1 large head cauliflower
1 cup shredded Mozzarella cheese
½ cup grated Parmesan cheese
1 large egg
¼ teaspoon garlic powder
¼ teaspoon dried parsley
⅛ teaspoon onion powder

1. On the stovetop, fill a large pot with 2 cups water and place a steamer in the pan. Bring water to a boil. Cut the cauliflower into florets and place on steamer basket. Cover pot with lid.
2. Allow cauliflower to steam 7 minutes until fork tender. Remove from steamer basket and place into cheesecloth or clean kitchen towel and let cool. Squeeze over sink to remove as much excess moisture as possible. The mixture will be too soft to form into tots if not all the moisture is removed. Mash with a fork to a smooth consistency.
3. Put the cauliflower into a large mixing bowl and add Mozzarella, Parmesan, egg, garlic powder, parsley, and onion powder. Stir until fully combined. The mixture should be wet but easy to mold.
4. Take 2 tablespoons of the mixture and roll into tot shape. Repeat with remaining mixture. Place into the air fryer basket.
5. Adjust the temperature to 320°F (160°C) and set the timer for 12 minutes.
6. Turn tots halfway through the cooking time. Cauliflower tots should be golden when fully cooked. Serve warm.

Per Serving
calories: 181 | fat: 9g | protein: 14g | carbs: 10g | net carbs: 7g | fiber: 3g

Cauliflower with Lime Juice

Prep time: 10 minutes | Cook time: 7 minutes | Serves 4

2 cups chopped cauliflower florets
2 tablespoons coconut oil, melted
2 teaspoons chili powder

½ teaspoon garlic powder

1 medium lime

2 tablespoons chopped cilantro

1. In a large bowl, toss cauliflower with coconut oil. Sprinkle with chili powder and garlic powder. Place seasoned cauliflower into the air fryer basket.
2. Adjust the temperature to 350°F (180ºC) and set the timer for 7 minutes.
3. Cauliflower will be tender and begin to turn golden at the edges. Place into serving bowl.
4. Cut the lime into quarters and squeeze juice over cauliflower. Garnish with cilantro.

Per Serving

calories: 73 | fat: 6g | protein: 1g | carbs: 3g | net carbs: 2g | fiber: 1g

Cheesy Cauliflower Rice Balls

Prep time: 10 minutes | Cook time: 8 minutes | Serves 4

1 (10-ounce / 283-g) steamer bag cauliflower rice, cooked according to package instructions

½ cup shredded Mozzarella cheese

1 large egg

2 ounces (57 g) plain pork rinds, finely crushed

¼ teaspoon salt

½ teaspoon Italian seasoning

1. Place cauliflower into a large bowl and mix with Mozzarella.
2. Whisk egg in a separate medium bowl. Place pork rinds into another large bowl with salt and Italian seasoning.
3. Separate cauliflower mixture into four equal sections and form each into a ball. Carefully dip a ball into whisked egg, then roll in pork rinds. Repeat with remaining balls.
4. Place cauliflower balls into ungreased air fryer basket. Adjust the temperature to 400°F (205ºC) and set the timer for 8 minutes. Rice balls will be golden when done.
5. Use a spatula to carefully move cauliflower balls to a large dish for serving. Serve warm.

Per Serving

calories: 158 | fat: 9g | protein: 15g | carbs: 4g | net carbs: 2g | fiber: 2g

Cheese Cauliflower Mash

Prep time: 10 minutes | Cook time: 15 minutes | Serves 6

1 (12-ounce / 340-g) steamer bag cauliflower florets, cooked according to package instructions

2 tablespoons salted butter, softened

2 ounces (57 g) cream cheese, softened

½ cup shredded sharp Cheddar cheese

¼ cup pickled jalapeños

½ teaspoon salt

¼ teaspoon ground black pepper

1. Place cooked cauliflower into a food processor with remaining ingredients. Pulse twenty times until cauliflower is smooth and all ingredients are combined.
2. Spoon mash into an ungreased 6-inch round nonstick baking dish. Place dish into air fryer basket. Adjust the temperature to 380°F (193ºC) and set the timer for 15 minutes. The top will be golden brown when done. Serve warm.

Per Serving

calories: 117 | fat: 9g | protein: 4g | carbs: 3g | net carbs: 2g | fiber: 1g

Broccoli with Sesame Dressing

Prep time: 5 minutes | Cook time: 10 minutes | Serves 4

6 cups broccoli florets, cut into bite-size pieces

1 tablespoon olive oil

¼ teaspoon salt

2 tablespoons sesame seeds

2 tablespoons rice vinegar

2 tablespoons coconut aminos

2 tablespoons sesame oil

½ teaspoon Swerve

¼ teaspoon red pepper flakes (optional)

1. Preheat the air fryer to 400°F (205ºC).

2. In a large bowl, toss the broccoli with the olive oil and salt until thoroughly coated.
3. Transfer the broccoli to the air fryer basket. Pausing halfway through the cooking time to shake the basket, air fry for 10 minutes until the stems are tender and the edges are beginning to crisp.
4. Meanwhile, in the same large bowl, whisk together the sesame seeds, vinegar, coconut aminos, sesame oil, Swerve, and red pepper flakes (if using).
5. Transfer the broccoli to the bowl and toss until thoroughly coated with the seasonings. Serve warm or at room temperature.

Per Serving

calories: 180 | fat: 13g | protein: 5g | carbs: 14g | net carbs: 10g | fiber: 4g

Cheesy Broccoli with Bacon

Prep time: 10 minutes | Cook time: 10 minutes | Serves 2

3 cups fresh broccoli florets

1 tablespoon coconut oil

½ cup shredded sharp Cheddar cheese

¼ cup full-fat sour cream

4 slices sugar-free bacon, cooked and crumbled

1 scallion, sliced on the bias

1. Place broccoli into the air fryer basket and drizzle it with coconut oil.
2. Adjust the temperature to 350°F (180°C) and set the timer for 10 minutes.
3. Toss the basket two or three times during cooking to avoid burned spots.
4. When broccoli begins to crisp at ends, remove from fryer. Top with shredded cheese, sour cream, and crumbled bacon and garnish with scallion slices.

Per Serving

calories: 361 | fat: 25g | protein: 18g | carbs: 11g | net carbs: 7g | fiber: 4g

Golden Broccoli Salad

Prep time: 5 minutes | Cook time: 7 minutes | Serves 4

2 cups fresh broccoli florets, chopped

1 tablespoon olive oil

¼ teaspoon salt

⅛ teaspoon ground black pepper

¼ cup lemon juice, divided

¼ cup shredded Parmesan cheese

¼ cup sliced roasted almonds

1. In a large bowl, toss broccoli and olive oil together. Sprinkle with salt and pepper, then drizzle with 2 tablespoons lemon juice.
2. Place broccoli into ungreased air fryer basket. Adjust the temperature to 350°F (180°C) and set the timer for 7 minutes, shaking the basket halfway through cooking. Broccoli will be golden on the edges when done.
3. Place broccoli into a large serving bowl and drizzle with remaining lemon juice. Sprinkle with Parmesan and almonds. Serve warm.

Per Serving

calories: 102 | fat: 7g | protein: 4g | carbs: 6g | net carbs: 4g | fiber: 2g

Tomato Salad with Arugula

Prep time: 10 minutes | Cook time: 10 minutes | Serves 4

4 green tomatoes

½ teaspoon salt

1 large egg, lightly beaten

½ cup peanut flour

1 tablespoon Creole seasoning

1 (5-ounce / 142-g) bag arugula

Buttermilk Dressing

1 cup mayonnaise

½ cup sour cream

2 teaspoons fresh lemon juice

2 tablespoons finely chopped fresh parsley

1 teaspoon dried dill

1 teaspoon dried chives

½ teaspoon salt

½ teaspoon garlic powder

½ teaspoon onion powder

1. Preheat the air fryer to 400°F (205ºC).
2. Slice the tomatoes into ½-inch slices and sprinkle with the salt. Let sit for 5 to 10 minutes.
3. Place the egg in a small shallow bowl. In another small shallow bowl, combine the peanut flour and Creole seasoning. Dip each tomato slice into the egg wash, then dip into the peanut flour mixture, turning to coat evenly.
4. Working in batches if necessary, arrange the tomato slices in a single layer in the air fryer basket and spray both sides lightly with olive oil. Air fry until browned and crisp, 8 to 10 minutes.
5. To make the buttermilk dressing: In a small bowl, whisk together the mayonnaise, sour cream, lemon juice, parsley, dill, chives, salt, garlic powder, and onion powder.
6. Serve the tomato slices on top of a bed of the arugula with the dressing on the side.

Per Serving

calories: 560 | fat: 54g | protein: 9g | carbs: 16g | net carbs: 13g | fiber: 3g

Air Fried Radishes

Prep time: 10 minutes | Cook time: 10 minutes | Serves 4

1 pound (454 g) radishes

2 tablespoons unsalted butter, melted

½ teaspoon garlic powder

½ teaspoon dried parsley

¼ teaspoon dried oregano

¼ teaspoon ground black pepper

1. Remove roots from radishes and cut into quarters.
2. In a small bowl, add butter and seasonings. Toss the radishes in the herb butter and place into the air fryer basket.
3. Adjust the temperature to 350°F (180ºC) and set the timer for 10 minutes.
4. Halfway through the cooking time, toss the radishes in the air fryer basket. Continue cooking until edges begin to turn brown.
5. Serve warm.

Per Serving

calories: 63 | fat: 5g | protein: 1g | carbs: 3g | net carbs: 2g | fiber: 1g

Sausage-Stuffed Mushroom Caps

Prep time: 10 minutes | Cook time: 8 minutes | Serves 2

6 large portobello mushroom caps

½ pound (227g) Italian sausage

¼ cup chopped onion

2 tablespoons blanched finely ground almond flour

¼ cup grated Parmesan cheese

1 teaspoon minced fresh garlic

1. Use a spoon to hollow out each mushroom cap, reserving scrapings.
2. In a medium skillet over medium heat, brown the sausage about 10 minutes or until fully cooked and no pink remains. Drain and then add reserved mushroom scrapings, onion, almond flour, Parmesan, and garlic. Gently fold ingredients together and continue cooking an additional minute, then remove from heat.
3. Evenly spoon the mixture into mushroom caps and place the caps into a 6-inch round pan. Place pan into the air fryer basket.
4. Adjust the temperature to 375°F (190ºC) and set the timer for 8 minutes.
5. When finished cooking, the tops will be browned and bubbling. Serve warm.

Per Serving

calories: 404 | fat: 25g | protein: 24g | carbs: 18g | net carbs: 14g | fiber: 4g

Air Fried Mushroom

Prep time: 10 minutes | Cook time: 10 minutes | Serves 4

8 ounces (227 g) cremini mushrooms, halved

2 tablespoons salted butter, melted

¼ teaspoon salt

¼ teaspoon ground black pepper

1. In a medium bowl, toss mushrooms with butter, then sprinkle with salt and pepper. Place into ungreased air fryer basket. Adjust the temperature to 400°F (205°C) and set the timer for 10 minutes, shaking the basket halfway through cooking. Mushrooms will be tender when done. Serve warm.

Per Serving

calories: 63 | fat: 5g | protein: 1g | carbs: 3g | net carbs: 3g | fiber: 0g

Roasted Eggplant

Prep time: 15 minutes | Cook time: 15 minutes | Serves 4

1 large eggplant

2 tablespoons olive oil

¼ teaspoon salt

½ teaspoon garlic powder

1. Remove top and bottom from eggplant. Slice eggplant into ¼-inch-thick round slices.
2. Brush slices with olive oil. Sprinkle with salt and garlic powder. Place eggplant slices into the air fryer basket.
3. Adjust the temperature to 390°F (199°C) and set the timer for 15 minutes.
4. Serve immediately.

Per Serving

calories: 236 | fat: 13g | protein: 19g | carbs: 5g | net carbs: 5g | fiber: 0g

Air Fried Cabbage

Prep time: 10 minutes | Cook time: 10 minutes | Serves 4

1 small head cabbage, cored and sliced into 1-inch-thick slices

2 tablespoons olive oil, divided

½ teaspoon salt

1 tablespoon Dijon mustard

1 teaspoon apple cider vinegar

1 teaspoon granular erythritol

1. Drizzle each cabbage slice with 1 tablespoon olive oil, then sprinkle with salt. Place slices into ungreased air fryer basket, working in batches if needed. Adjust the temperature to 350°F (180°C) and set the timer for 10 minutes. Cabbage will be tender and edges will begin to brown when done.
2. In a small bowl, whisk remaining olive oil with mustard, vinegar, and erythritol. Drizzle over cabbage in a large serving dish. Serve warm.

Per Serving

calories: 111 | fat: 7g | protein: 3g | carbs: 12g | net carbs: 8g | fiber: 4g

Pork and Onion Rings

Prep time: 10 minutes | Cook time: 5 minutes | Serves 8

1 large egg
¼ cup coconut flour
2 ounces (57 g) plain pork rinds, finely crushed
1 large white onion, peeled and sliced into 8 (¼-inch) rings

1. Whisk egg in a medium bowl. Place coconut flour and pork rinds in two separate medium bowls. Dip each onion ring into egg, then coat in coconut flour. Dip coated onion ring in egg once more, then press gently into pork rinds to cover all sides.
2. Place rings into ungreased air fryer basket. Adjust the temperature to 400°F (205°C) and set the timer for 5 minutes, turning the onion rings halfway through cooking. Onion rings will be golden and crispy when done. Serve warm.

Per Serving

calories: 79 | fat: 3g | protein: 6g | carbs: 6g | net carbs: 4g | fiber: 2g

Cheesy Spinach Poppers

Prep time: 10 minutes | Cook time: 8 minutes | Makes 16 poppers

4 ounces (113 g) cream cheese, softened
1 cup chopped fresh spinach leaves

½ teaspoon garlic powder

8 mini sweet bell peppers, tops removed, seeded, and halved lengthwise

1. In a medium bowl, mix cream cheese, spinach, and garlic powder. Place 1 tablespoon mixture into each sweet pepper half and press down to smooth.
2. Place poppers into ungreased air fryer basket. Adjust the temperature to 400°F (205ºC) and set the timer for 8 minutes. Poppers will be done when cheese is browned on top and peppers are tender-crisp. Serve warm.

Per Serving

calories: 116 | fat: 8g | protein: 3g | carbs: 5g | net carbs: 4g | fiber: 1g

Roasted Salsa

Prep time: 5 minutes | Cook time: 30 minutes | Makes 2 cups

2 large San Marzano tomatoes, cored and cut into large chunks

½ medium white onion, peeled and large-diced

½ medium jalapeño, seeded and large-diced

2 cloves garlic, peeled and diced

½ teaspoon salt

1 tablespoon coconut oil

¼ cup fresh lime juice

1. Place tomatoes, onion, and jalapeño into an ungreased 6-inch round nonstick baking dish. Add garlic, then sprinkle with salt and drizzle with coconut oil.
2. Place dish into air fryer basket. Adjust the temperature to 300°F (150ºC) and set the timer for 30 minutes. Vegetables will be dark brown around the edges and tender when done.
3. Pour mixture into a food processor or blender. Add lime juice. Process on low speed 30 seconds until only a few chunks remain.
4. Transfer salsa to a sealable container and refrigerate at least 1 hour. Serve chilled.

Per Serving

calories: 28 | fat: 2g | protein: 1g | carbs: 3g | net carbs: 2g | fiber: 1g

Vegetarian Mains

Cheesy Eggplant Lasagna

Prep time: 15 minutes | Cook time: 36 minutes | Serves 4

1 small eggplant (about ¾ pound / 340 g), sliced into rounds

2 teaspoons salt

1 tablespoon olive oil

1 cup shredded Mozzarella, divided

1 cup ricotta cheese

1 large egg

¼ cup grated Parmesan cheese

½ teaspoon dried oregano

1½ cups no-sugar-added marinara

1 tablespoon chopped fresh parsley

1. Preheat the air fryer to 350°F (180ºC). Coat a 6-cup casserole dish that fits in your air fryer with olive oil; set aside.
2. Arrange the eggplant slices in a single layer on a baking sheet and sprinkle with the salt. Let sit for 10 minutes. Use a paper towel to remove the excess moisture and salt.
3. Working in batches if necessary, brush the eggplant with the olive oil and arrange in a single layer in the air fryer basket. Pausing halfway through the cooking time to turn the eggplant, air fry for 6 minutes until softened. Transfer the eggplant back to the baking sheet and let cool.
4. In a small bowl, combine ½ cup of the Mozzarella with the ricotta, egg, Parmesan, and oregano. To assemble the lasagna, spread a spoonful of marinara in the bottom of the casserole dish, followed by a layer of eggplant, a layer of the cheese mixture, and a layer of marinara. Repeat the layers until all of the ingredients are used, ending with the remaining ½ cup of Mozzarella. Scatter the parsley on top. Cover the baking dish with foil.
5. Increase the air fryer to 370°F (188ºC) and air fry for 30 minutes. Uncover the dish and continue baking for 10 minutes longer until the cheese begins to brown. Let the casserole sit for at least 10 minutes before serving.

Per Serving

calories: 350 | fat: 22g | protein: 20g | carbs: 17g | net carbs: 12g | fiber: 5g

Zucchini Cheese Tart

Prep time: 15 minutes | Cook time: 50 minutes | Serves 6

½ cup grated Parmesan cheese, divided

1½ cups almond flour

1 tablespoon coconut flour

½ teaspoon garlic powder

¾ teaspoon salt, divided

¼ cup unsalted butter, melted

1 zucchini, thinly sliced (about 2 cups)

1 cup ricotta cheese

3 eggs

2 tablespoons heavy cream

2 cloves garlic, minced

½ teaspoon dried tarragon

1. Preheat the air fryer to 330°F (166°C). Coat a round 6-cup pan with olive oil and set aside.
2. In a large bowl, whisk ¼ cup of the Parmesan with the almond flour, coconut flour, garlic powder, and ¼ teaspoon of the salt. Stir in the melted butter until the dough resembles coarse crumbs. Press the dough firmly into the bottom and up the sides of the prepared pan. Air fry for 12 to 15 minutes until the crust begins to brown. Let cool to room temperature.
3. Meanwhile, place the zucchini in a colander and sprinkle with the remaining ½ teaspoon salt. Toss gently to distribute the salt and let sit for 30 minutes. Use paper towels to pat the zucchini dry.
4. In a large bowl, whisk together the ricotta, eggs, heavy cream, garlic, and tarragon. Gently stir in the zucchini slices. Pour the cheese mixture into the cooled crust and sprinkle with the remaining ¼ cup Parmesan.
5. Increase the air fryer to 350°F (180°C). Place the pan in the air fryer basket and air fry for 45 to 50 minutes, or until set and a tester inserted into the center of the tart comes out clean. Serve warm or at room temperature.

Per Serving

calories: 390 | fat: 30g | protein: 19g | carbs: 14g | net carbs: 12g | fiber: 2g

Cauliflower with Cheese

Prep time: 15 minutes | Cook time: 30 minutes | Serve: 4

5 cups cauliflower florets

2/3 cup almond flour

½ teaspoon salt

¼ cup unsalted butter, melted

¼ cup grated Parmesan cheese

1. In a food processor fitted with a metal blade, pulse the cauliflower until finely chopped. Transfer the cauliflower to a large microwave-safe bowl and cover it with a paper towel. Microwave for 5 minutes. Spread the cauliflower on a towel to cool.
2. When cool enough to handle, draw up the sides of the towel and squeeze tightly over a sink to remove the excess moisture. Return the cauliflower to the food processor and whirl until creamy. Sprinkle in the flour and salt and pulse until a sticky dough comes together.
3. Transfer the dough to a workspace lightly floured with almond flour. Shape the dough into a ball and divide into 4 equal sections. Roll each section into a rope 1-inch thick. Slice the dough into squares with a sharp knife.
4. Preheat the air fryer to 400°F (205°C).
5. Working in batches if necessary, place the gnocchi in a single layer in the basket of the air fryer and spray generously with olive oil. Pausing halfway through the cooking time to turn the gnocchi, air fry for 25 to 30 minutes until golden brown and crispy on the edges. Transfer to a large bowl and toss with the melted butter and Parmesan cheese.

Per Serving

calories: 360 | fat: 20g | protein: 9g | carbs: 14g | net carbs: 10g | fiber: 4g

Cauliflower Steak With Gremolata

Prep time: 15 minutes | Cook time: 25 minutes | Serves 4

2 tablespoons olive oil

1 tablespoon Italian seasoning

1 large head cauliflower, outer leaves removed and sliced lengthwise through the core into thick "steaks"

Salt and freshly ground black pepper

¼ cup Parmesan cheese

Gremolata :

1 bunch Italian parsley (about 1 cup packed)

2 cloves garlic

Zest of 1 small lemon, plus 1–2 teaspoons lemon juice

½ cup olive oil

Salt and pepper to taste

1. Preheat the air fryer to 400°F (205ºC).
2. In a small bowl, combine the olive oil and Italian seasoning. Brush both sides of each cauliflower "steak" generously with the oil. Season to taste with salt and black pepper.
3. Working in batches if necessary, arrange the cauliflower in a single layer in the air fryer basket. Pausing halfway through the cooking time to turn the "steaks," air fry for 15 to 20 minutes until the cauliflower is tender and the edges begin to brown. Sprinkle with the Parmesan and air fry for 5 minutes longer.
4. To make the gremolata: In a food processor fitted with a metal blade, combine the parsley, garlic, and lemon zest and juice. With the motor running, add the olive oil in a steady stream until the mixture forms a bright green sauce. Season to taste with salt and black pepper. Serve the cauliflower steaks with the gremolata spooned over the top.

Per Serving

calories: 390 | fat: 36g | protein: 7g | carbs: 14g | net carbs: 8g | fiber: 6g

Broccoli-Cheese Fritters

Prep time: 10 minutes | Cook time: 25 minutes | Serves 4

1 cup broccoli florets

1 cup shredded Mozzarella cheese

¾ cup almond flour

½ cup flaxseed meal, divided

2 teaspoons baking powder

1 teaspoon garlic powder

Salt and freshly ground black pepper

2 eggs, lightly beaten

½ cup ranch dressing

1. Preheat the air fryer to 400°F (205ºC).
2. In a food processor fitted with a metal blade, pulse the broccoli until very finely chopped.

3. Transfer the broccoli to a large bowl and add the Mozzarella, almond flour, ¼ cup of the flaxseed meal, baking powder, and garlic powder. Stir until thoroughly combined. Season to taste with salt and black pepper. Add the eggs and stir again to form a sticky dough. Shape the dough into 1¼-inch fritters.
4. Place the remaining ¼ cup flaxseed meal in a shallow bowl and roll the fritters in the meal to form an even coating.
5. Working in batches if necessary, arrange the fritters in a single layer in the basket of the air fryer and spray generously with olive oil. Pausing halfway through the cooking time to shake the basket, air fry for 20 to 25 minutes until the fritters are golden brown and crispy. Serve with the ranch dressing for dipping.

Per Serving

calories: 450 | fat: 36g | protein: 19g | carbs: 16g | net carbs: 10g | fiber: 6g

Air Fried Tofu

Prep time: 10 minutes | Cook time: 20 minutes | Serves 4

1 (16-ounce / 454-g) block extra-firm tofu

2 tablespoons coconut aminos

1 tablespoon toasted sesame oil

1 tablespoon olive oil

1 tablespoon chili-garlic sauce

1½ teaspoons black sesame seeds

1 scallion, thinly sliced

1. Press the tofu for at least 15 minutes by wrapping it in paper towels and setting a heavy pan on top so that the moisture drains.
2. Slice the tofu into bite-size cubes and transfer to a bowl. Drizzle with the coconut aminos, sesame oil, olive oil, and chili-garlic sauce. Cover and refrigerate for 1 hour or up to overnight.
3. Preheat the air fryer to 400°F (205°C).
4. Arrange the tofu in a single layer in the air fryer basket. Pausing to shake the pan halfway through the cooking time, air fry for 15 to 20 minutes until crisp. Serve with any juices that accumulate in the bottom of the air fryer, sprinkled with the sesame seeds and sliced scallion.

Per Serving

calories: 180 | fat: 13g | protein: 11g | carbs: 5g | net carbs: 4g | fiber: 1g

Cheesy Mushroom Soufflés

Prep time: 15 minutes | Cook time: 12 minutes | Serves 4

3 large eggs, whites and yolks separated

½ cup sharp white Cheddar cheese

3 ounces (85 g) cream cheese, softened

¼ teaspoon cream of tartar

¼ teaspoon salt

¼ teaspoon ground black pepper

½ cup cremini mushrooms, sliced

1. In a large bowl, whip egg whites until stiff peaks form, about 2 minutes. In a separate large bowl, beat Cheddar, egg yolks, cream cheese, cream of tartar, salt, and pepper together until combined.
2. Fold egg whites into cheese mixture, being careful not to stir. Fold in mushrooms, then pour mixture evenly into four ungreased 4-inch ramekins.
3. Place ramekins into air fryer basket. Adjust the temperature to 350°F (180ºC) and set the timer for 12 minutes. Eggs will be browned on the top and firm in the center when done. Serve warm.

Per Serving

calories: 185 | fat: 14g | protein: 10g | carbs: 2g | net carbs: 2g | fiber: 0g

Spinach Cheese Casserole

Prep time: 15 minutes | Cook time: 15 minutes | Serves 4

1 tablespoon salted butter, melted

¼ cup diced yellow onion

8 ounces (227 g) full-fat cream cheese, softened

⅓ cup full-fat mayonnaise

⅓ cup full-fat sour cream

¼ cup chopped pickled jalapeños

2 cups fresh spinach, chopped

2 cups cauliflower florets, chopped

1 cup artichoke hearts, chopped

1. In a large bowl, mix butter, onion, cream cheese, mayonnaise, and sour cream. Fold in jalapeños, spinach, cauliflower, and artichokes.
2. Pour the mixture into a 4-cup round baking dish. Cover with foil and place into the air fryer basket.
3. Adjust the temperature to 370°F (188ºC) and set the timer for 15 minutes.
4. In the last 2 minutes of cooking, remove the foil to brown the top. Serve warm.

Per Serving

calories: 423 | fat: 36.3g | protein: 6.7g | carbs: 12.1g | net carbs: 6.8g | fiber: 5.3g

Roasted Spaghetti Squash

Prep time: 10 minutes | Cook time: 45 minutes | Serves 6

1 (4-pound / 1.8-kg) spaghetti squash, halved and seeded

2 tablespoons coconut oil

4 tablespoons salted butter, melted

1 teaspoon garlic powder

2 teaspoons dried parsley

1. Brush shell of spaghetti squash with coconut oil. Brush inside with butter. Sprinkle inside with garlic powder and parsley.
2. Place squash skin side down into ungreased air fryer basket, working in batches if needed. Adjust the temperature to 350°F (180ºC) and set the timer for 30 minutes. When the timer beeps, flip squash and cook an additional 15 minutes until fork-tender.
3. Use a fork to remove spaghetti strands from shell and serve warm.

Per Serving

calories: 104 | fat: 7g | protein: 1g | carbs: 9g | net carbs: 7g | fiber: 2g

Cheesy Zucchini

Prep time: 10 minutes | Cook time: 8 minutes | Serves 4

2 tablespoons salted butter

¼ cup diced white onion

½ teaspoon minced garlic

½ cup heavy whipping cream

2 ounces (57 g) full-fat cream cheese

1 cup shredded sharp Cheddar cheese

2 medium zucchini, spiralized

1. In a large saucepan over medium heat, melt butter. Add onion and sauté until it begins to soften, 1–3 minutes. Add garlic and sauté 30 seconds, then pour in cream and add cream cheese.
2. Remove the pan from heat and stir in Cheddar. Add the zucchini and toss in the sauce, then put into a 4-cup round baking dish. Cover the dish with foil and place into the air fryer basket.
3. Adjust the temperature to 370°F (188°C) and set the timer for 8 minutes.
4. After 6 minutes remove the foil and let the top brown for remaining cooking time. Stir and serve.

Per Serving

calories: 337 | fat: 28.4g | protein: 9.6g | carbs: 5.9g | net carbs: 4.7g | fiber: 1.2g

Zucchini and Mushroom Kebab

Prep time: 40 minutes | Cook time: 8 minutes | Makes 8 skewers

1 medium zucchini, trimmed and cut into ½-inch slices

½ medium yellow onion, peeled and cut into 1-inch squares

1 medium red bell pepper, seeded and cut into 1-inch squares

16 whole cremini mushrooms

⅓ cup basil pesto

½ teaspoon salt

¼ teaspoon ground black pepper

1. Divide zucchini slices, onion, and bell pepper into eight even portions. Place on 6-inch skewers for a total of eight kebabs. Add 2 mushrooms to each skewer and brush kebabs generously with pesto.

2. Sprinkle each kebab with salt and black pepper on all sides, then place into ungreased air fryer basket. Adjust the temperature to 375°F (190ºC) and set the timer for 8 minutes, turning kebabs halfway through cooking. Vegetables will be browned at the edges and tender-crisp when done. Serve warm.

Per Serving

calories: 107 | fat: 7g | protein: 4g | carbs: 10g | net carbs: 8g | fiber: 2g

Eggplant with Tomato and Cheese

Prep time: 35 minutes | Cook time: 5 minutes | Serves 4

1 eggplant, peeled and sliced

2 bell peppers, seeded and sliced

1 red onion, sliced

1 teaspoon fresh garlic, minced

4 tablespoons olive oil

1 teaspoon mustard

1 teaspoon dried oregano

1 teaspoon smoked paprika

Salt and ground black pepper, to taste

1 tomato, sliced

6 ounces (170 g) halloumi cheese, sliced lengthways

1. Start by preheating your Air Fryer to 370 degrees F (188ºC). Spritz a baking pan with nonstick cooking spray.
2. Place the eggplant, peppers, onion, and garlic on the bottom of the baking pan. Add the olive oil, mustard, and spices. Transfer to the cooking basket and cook for 14 minutes.
3. Top with the tomatoes and cheese; increase the temperature to 390 degrees F (199ºC) and cook for 5 minutes more until bubbling. Let it sit on a cooling rack for 10 minutes before serving.
4. Bon appétit!

Per Serving

calories: 306 | fat: 16.1g | protein: 39.6g | carbs: 8.8g | net carbs: 7g | fiber: 1.8g

Roast Eggplant and Zucchini Bites

Prep time: 35 minutes | Cook time: 30 minutes | Serves 8

2 teaspoons fresh mint leaves, chopped

1½ teaspoons red pepper chili flakes

2 tablespoons melted butter

1 pound (454 g) eggplant, peeled and cubed

1 pound (454 g) zucchini, peeled and cubed

3 tablespoons olive oil

1. Toss all of the above ingredients in a large-sized mixing dish.
2. Roast the eggplant and zucchini bites for 30 minutes at 325 degrees F (163ºC) in your Air Fryer, turning once or twice.
3. Serve with a homemade dipping sauce.

Per Serving

calories: 110 | fat: 8.3g | protein: 2.6g | carbs: 8.8g | net carbs: 6.3g | fiber: 2.5g

Cheesy Zucchini and Spinach

Prep time: 9 minutes | Cook time: 7 minutes | Serves 6

4 eggs, slightly beaten

1/2 cup almond flour

1/2 cup goat cheese, crumbled

1 teaspoon fine sea salt

4 garlic cloves, minced

1 cup baby spinach

1/2 cup Parmesan cheese grated

1/3 teaspoon red pepper flakes

1 pound (454 g) zucchini, peeled and grated

1/3 teaspoon dried dill weed

1. Thoroughly combine all ingredients in a bowl. Now, roll the mixture to form small croquettes.
2. Air fry at 335 degrees F (168ºC) for 7 minutes or until golden. Tate, adjust for seasonings and serve warm.

Per Serving

calories: 171 | fat: 10.8g | protein: 3.1g | carbs: 15.9g | net carbs: 14.9g | fiber: 1g

Cheese Stuffed Zucchini

Prep time: 20 minutes | Cook time: 8 minutes | Serves 4

1 large zucchini, cut into four pieces

2 tablespoons olive oil

1 cup Ricotta cheese, room temperature

2 tablespoons scallions, chopped

1 heaping tablespoon fresh parsley, roughly chopped

1 heaping tablespoon coriander, minced

2 ounces (57 g) Cheddar cheese, preferably freshly grated

1 teaspoon celery seeds

½ teaspoon salt

½ teaspoon garlic pepper

1. Cook your zucchini in the Air Fryer cooking basket for approximately 10 minutes at 350 degrees F (180ºC). Check for doneness and cook for 2-3 minutes longer if needed.
2. Meanwhile, make the stuffing by mixing the other items.
3. When your zucchini is thoroughly cooked, open them up. Divide the stuffing among all zucchini pieces and bake an additional 5 minutes.

Per Serving

calories: 199 | fat: 16.4g | protein: 9.2g | carbs: 4.5g | net carbs: 4g | fiber: 0.5g

Cheese Stuffed Pepper

Prep time: 20 minutes | Cook time: 15 minutes | Serves 2

1 red bell pepper, top and seeds removed

1 yellow bell pepper, top and seeds removed

Salt and pepper, to taste

1 cup Cottage cheese

4 tablespoons mayonnaise

2 pickles, chopped

1. Arrange the peppers in the lightly greased cooking basket. Cook in the preheated Air Fryer at 400 degrees F (205ºC) for 15 minutes, turning them over halfway through the cooking time.
2. Season with salt and pepper.
3. Then, in a mixing bowl, combine the cream cheese with the mayonnaise and chopped pickles. Stuff the pepper with the cream cheese mixture and serve. Enjoy!

Per Serving

calories: 360 | fat: 27.3g | protein: 20.3g | carbs: 7.6g | net carbs: 6.4g | fiber: 1.2g

Air Fried Cheesy Mushroom

Prep time: 10 minutes | Cook time: 14 minutes | Serves 4

2 tablespoons olive oil

4 large portobello mushrooms, stems removed and gills scraped out

½ teaspoon salt

¼ teaspoon freshly ground pepper

4 ounces (113 g) goat cheese, crumbled

½ cup chopped marinated artichoke hearts

1 cup frozen spinach, thawed and squeezed dry

½ cup grated Parmesan cheese

2 tablespoons chopped fresh parsley

1. Preheat the air fryer to 400°F (205ºC).
2. Rub the olive oil over the portobello mushrooms until thoroughly coated. Sprinkle both sides with the salt and black pepper. Place top-side down on a clean work surface.
3. In a small bowl, combine the goat cheese, artichoke hearts, and spinach. Mash with the back of a fork until thoroughly combined. Divide the cheese mixture among the mushrooms and sprinkle with the Parmesan cheese.

4. Air fry for 10 to 14 minutes until the mushrooms are tender and the cheese has begun to brown. Top with the fresh parsley just before serving.

Per Serving

calories: 270 | fat: 23g | protein: 8g | carbs: 11g | net carbs: 7g | fiber: 4g

Cheesy Celery Croquettes with Chive Mayo

Prep time: 15 minutes | Cook time: 6 minutes | Serves 4

2 medium-sized celery stalks, trimmed and grated

½ cup of leek, finely chopped

1 tablespoon garlic paste

¼ teaspoon freshly cracked black pepper

1 teaspoon fine sea salt

1 tablespoon fresh dill, finely chopped

1 egg, lightly whisked

¼ cup almond flour

½ cup Parmesan cheese, freshly grated

¼ teaspoon baking powder

2 tablespoons fresh chives, chopped

4 tablespoons mayonnaise

1. Place the celery on a paper towel and squeeze them to remove excess liquid.
2. Combine the vegetables with the other ingredients, except the chives and mayo. Shape the balls using 1 tablespoon of the vegetable mixture.
3. Then, gently flatten each ball with your palm or a wide spatula. Spritz the croquettes with a non - stick cooking oil.
4. Air-fry the vegetable croquettes in a single layer for 6 minutes at 360 degrees F (182ºC).
5. Meanwhile, mix fresh chives and mayonnaise. Serve warm croquettes with chive mayo. Bon appétit!

Per Serving

calories: 214 | fat: 18g | protein: 7g | carbs: 6.8g | net carbs: 5.2g | fiber: 1.6g

Cauliflower Cheese Fritters

Prep time: 15 minutes | Cook time: 10 minutes | Serves 8

2 pounds (907 g) cauliflower florets

½ cup scallions, finely chopped

½ teaspoon freshly ground black pepper, or more to taste

1 tablespoon fine sea salt

½ teaspoon hot paprika

2 cups Colby cheese, shredded

1 cup Parmesan cheese, grated

¼ cup olive oil

1. Firstly, boil the cauliflower until fork tender. Drain, peel and mash your cauliflower.
2. Thoroughly mix the mashed cauliflower with scallions, pepper, salt, paprika, and Colby cheese. Then, shape the balls using your hands. Now, flatten the balls to make the patties.
3. Roll the patties over grated Parmesan cheese. Drizzle olive oil over them.
4. Next, cook your patties at 360 degrees F (182ºC) approximately 10 minutes, working in batches. Serve with tabasco mayo if desired. Bon appétit!

Per Serving

calories: 282 | fat: 22g | protein: 13g | carbs: 8g | net carbs: 6g | fiber: 2g

Broccoli with Garlic Sauce

Prep time: 19 minutes | Cook time: 15 minutes | Serves 4

2 tablespoons olive oil

Kosher salt and freshly ground black pepper, to taste

1 pound (454 g) broccoli florets

For the Dipping Sauce:

2 teaspoons dried rosemary, crushed

3 garlic cloves, minced

$1/3$ teaspoon dried marjoram, crushed

¼ cup sour cream

$1/3$ cup mayonnaise

1. Lightly grease your broccoli with a thin layer of olive oil. Season with salt and ground black pepper.
2. Arrange the seasoned broccoli in an Air Fryer cooking basket. Bake at 395 degrees F (202ºC) for 15 minutes, shaking once or twice.
3. In the meantime, prepare the dipping sauce by mixing all the sauce ingredients. Serve warm broccoli with the dipping sauce and enjoy!

Per Serving

calories: 247 | fat: 22g | protein: 4g | carbs: 9g | net carbs: 6g | fiber: 3g

Air Fried Asparagus and Broccoli

Prep time: 25 minutes | Cook time: 22 minutes | Serves 4

½ pound (227g) asparagus, cut into 1 ½-inch pieces

½ pound (227g) broccoli, cut into 1 ½-inch pieces

2 tablespoons olive oil

Some salt and white pepper, to taste

½ cup vegetable broth

2 tablespoons apple cider vinegar

1. Place the vegetables in a single layer in the lightly greased cooking basket. Drizzle the olive oil over the vegetables.
2. Sprinkle with salt and white pepper.
3. Cook at 380 degrees F (193ºC) for 15 minutes, shaking the basket halfway through the cooking time.
4. Add ½ cup of vegetable broth to a saucepan; bring to a rapid boil and add the vinegar. Cook for 5 to 7 minutes or until the sauce has reduced by half.
5. Spoon the sauce over the warm vegetables and serve immediately. Bon appétit!

Per Serving

calories: 181 | fat: 7g | protein: 3g | carbs: 4g | net carbs: 1g | fiber: 3g

Poultry

Chicken with Lettuce

Prep time: 15 minutes | Cook time: 14 minutes | Serves 4

1 pound (454 g) chicken breast tenders, chopped into bite-size pieces
½ onion, thinly sliced
½ red bell pepper, seeded and thinly sliced
½ green bell pepper, seeded and thinly sliced
1 tablespoon olive oil
1 tablespoon fajita seasoning
1 teaspoon kosher salt
Juice of ½ lime
8 large lettuce leaves
1 cup prepared guacamole

1. Preheat the air fryer to 400°F (205ºC).
2. In a large bowl, combine the chicken, onion, and peppers. Drizzle with the olive oil and toss until thoroughly coated. Add the fajita seasoning and salt and toss again.
3. Working in batches if necessary, arrange the chicken and vegetables in a single layer in the air fryer basket. Pausing halfway through the cooking time to shake the basket, air fry for 14 minutes, or until the vegetables are tender and a thermometer inserted into the thickest piece of chicken registers 165°F (74ºC).
4. Transfer the mixture to a serving platter and drizzle with the fresh lime juice. Serve with the lettuce leaves and top with the guacamole.

Per Serving

calories: 330 | fat: 22g | protein: 25g | carbs: 8g | net carbs: 3g | fiber: 5g

Bacon Chicken Salad

Prep time: 15 minutes | Cook time: 8 minutes | Serves 4

8 slices reduced-sodium bacon

8 chicken breast tenders (about 1½ pounds / 680g)

8 cups chopped romaine lettuce

1 cup cherry tomatoes, halved

¼ red onion, thinly sliced

2 hard-boiled eggs, peeled and sliced

Avocado-Lime Dressing:

½ cup plain Greek yogurt

¼ cup milk

½ avocado

Juice of ½ lime

3 scallions, coarsely chopped

1 clove garlic

2 tablespoons fresh cilantro

⅛ teaspoon ground cumin

Salt and freshly ground black pepper

1. Preheat the air fryer to 400°F (205°C).
2. Wrap a piece of bacon around each piece of chicken and secure with a toothpick. Working in batches if necessary, arrange the bacon-wrapped chicken in a single layer in the air fryer basket. Air fry for 8 minutes until the bacon is browned and a thermometer inserted into the thickest piece of chicken register 165°F (74°C). Let cool for a few minutes, then slice into bite-size pieces.
3. To make the dressing: In a blender or food processor, combine the yogurt, milk, avocado, lime juice, scallions, garlic, cilantro, and cumin. purée until smooth. Season to taste with salt and freshly ground pepper.
4. To assemble the salad, in a large bowl, combine the lettuce, tomatoes, and onion. Drizzle the dressing over the vegetables and toss gently until thoroughly combined. Arrange the chicken and eggs on top just before serving.

Per Serving

calories: 425 | fat: 18g | protein: 52g | carbs: 11g | net carbs: 7g | fiber: 4g

Lemon Chicken

Prep time: 10 minutes | Cook time: 25 minutes | Serves 4

8 bone-in chicken thighs, skin on

1 tablespoon olive oil

1½ teaspoons lemon-pepper seasoning

½ teaspoon paprika

½ teaspoon garlic powder

¼ teaspoon freshly ground black pepper

Juice of ½ lemon

1. Preheat the air fryer to 360°F (182ºC).
2. Place the chicken in a large bowl and drizzle with the olive oil. Top with the lemon-pepper seasoning, paprika, garlic powder, and freshly ground black pepper. Toss until thoroughly coated.
3. Working in batches if necessary, arrange the chicken in a single layer in the basket of the air fryer. Pausing halfway through the cooking time to turn the chicken, air fry for 20 to 25 minutes, until a thermometer inserted into the thickest piece registers 165°F (74ºC).
4. Transfer the chicken to a serving platter and squeeze the lemon juice over the top.

Per Serving

calories: 335 | fat: 22g | protein: 31g | carbs: 0g | net carbs: 0g | fiber:0g

Savory Chicken

Prep time: 5 minutes | Cook time: 13 to 16 minutes | Serves 6

½ cup sugar-free mayonnaise (homemade, [here](), or store-bought)

1 tablespoon Dijon mustard

1 tablespoon freshly squeezed lemon juice (optional)

1 tablespoon coconut aminos

1 teaspoon Italian seasoning

1 teaspoon sea salt

½ teaspoon freshly ground black pepper

¼ teaspoon cayenne pepper

1½ pounds (680g) boneless, skinless chicken breasts or thighs

1. In a small bowl, combine the mayonnaise, mustard, lemon juice (if using), coconut aminos, Italian seasoning, salt, black pepper, and cayenne pepper.
2. Place the chicken in a shallow dish or large zip-top plastic bag. Add the marinade, making sure all the pieces are coated. Cover and refrigerate for at least 30 minutes or up to 4 hours.
3. Set the air fryer to 400°F (205°C). Arrange the chicken in a single layer in the air fryer basket, working in batches if necessary. Cook for 7 minutes. Flip the chicken and continue cooking for 6 to 9 minutes more, until an instant-read thermometer reads 160°F (71°C).

Per Serving

calories: 236 | fat: 17g | protein: 23g | carbs: 2g | net carbs: 1g | fiber: 1g

Chicken Thighs with Cilantro

Prep time: 15 minutes | Cook time: 25 minutes | Serves 4

1 tablespoon olive oil

Juice of ½ lime

1 tablespoon coconut aminos

1½ teaspoons Montreal chicken seasoning

8 bone-in chicken thighs, skin on

2 tablespoons chopped fresh cilantro

1. In a gallon-size resealable bag, combine the olive oil, lime juice, coconut aminos, and chicken seasoning. Add the chicken thighs, seal the bag, and massage the bag to ensure the chicken is thoroughly coated. Refrigerate for at least 2 hours, preferably overnight.
2. Preheat the air fryer to 400°F (205°C).
3. Remove the chicken from the marinade (discard the marinade) and arrange in a single layer in the air fryer basket. Pausing halfway through the cooking time to flip the chicken, air fry for 20 to 25 minutes, until a thermometer inserted into the thickest part registers 165°F (74°C).
4. Transfer the chicken to a serving platter and top with the cilantro before serving.

Per Serving

calories: 335 | fat: 22g | protein: 31g | carbs: 0g | net carbs: 0g | fiber: 0g

Air Fried Chicken

Prep time: 15 minutes | Cook time: 20 minutes | Serves 6

2 teaspoons ground coriander

1 teaspoon ground allspice

1 teaspoon cayenne pepper

1 teaspoon ground ginger

1 teaspoon salt

1 teaspoon dried thyme

½ teaspoon ground cinnamon

½ teaspoon ground nutmeg

2 pounds (907 g) boneless chicken thighs, skin on

2 tablespoons olive oil

1. In a small bowl, combine the coriander, allspice, cayenne, ginger, salt, thyme, cinnamon, and nutmeg. Stir until thoroughly combined.
2. Place the chicken in a 9 × 13-inch baking dish and use paper towels to pat dry. Thoroughly coat both sides of the chicken with the spice mixture. Cover and refrigerate for at least 2 hours, preferably overnight.
3. Preheat the air fryer to 360°F (182°C).
4. Working in batches if necessary, arrange the chicken in a single layer in the air fryer basket and lightly coat with the olive oil. Pausing halfway through the cooking time to flip the chicken, air fry for 15 to 20 minutes, until a thermometer inserted into the thickest part registers 165°F (74°C).

Per Serving

calories: 223 | fat: 11g | protein: 30g | carbs: 1g | net carbs: 1g | fiber: 0g

Aromatic Chicken

Prep time: 15 minutes | Cook time: 30 minutes | Serves 4

1 (4-pound / 1.8 kg) chicken, giblets removed

½ onion, quartered

1 tablespoon olive oil

Secret Spice Rub

2 teaspoons salt

1 teaspoon paprika

½ teaspoon onion powder

½ teaspoon garlic powder

½ teaspoon dried thyme

½ teaspoon freshly ground black pepper

¼ teaspoon cayenne

1. Preheat the air fryer to 350°F (180ºC).
2. Use paper towels to blot the chicken dry. Stuff the chicken with the onion. Rub the chicken with the oil.
3. To make the spice rub: In a small bowl, combine the salt, paprika, onion powder, garlic powder, thyme, black pepper, and cayenne; stir until thoroughly combined. Sprinkle the chicken with the spice rub until thoroughly coated.
4. Place the chicken breast side down in the air fryer basket. Air fry the chicken for 30 minutes. Use tongs to carefully flip the chicken over and air fry for an additional 30 minutes, or until the temperature of a thermometer inserted into the thickest part of the chicken registers 165°F (74ºC).
5. Let the chicken rest for 10 minutes. Discard the onion and serve.

Per Serving

calories: 500 | fat: 27g | protein: 61g | carbs: 2g | net carbs: 0g | fiber: 2g

Cheesy Chicken Breast

Prep time: 15 minutes | Cook time: 25 minutes | Serves 4

4 small boneless, skinless chicken breast halves (about 1½ pounds / 680g)

Salt and freshly ground black pepper

4 ounces (113 g) goat cheese

6 pitted Kalamata olives, coarsely chopped

Zest of ½ lemon

1 teaspoon minced fresh rosemary or ½ teaspoon ground dried rosemary

½ cup almond meal

¼ cup balsamic vinegar

6 tablespoons unsalted butter

1. Preheat the air fryer to 360°F (182°C).
2. With a boning knife, cut a wide pocket into the thickest part of each chicken breast half, taking care not to cut all the way through. Season the chicken evenly on both sides with salt and freshly ground black pepper.
3. In a small bowl, mix the cheese, olives, lemon zest, and rosemary. Stuff the pockets with the cheese mixture and secure with toothpicks.
4. Place the almond meal in a shallow bowl and dredge the chicken, shaking off the excess. Coat lightly with olive oil spray.
5. Working in batches if necessary, arrange the chicken breasts in a single layer in the air fryer basket. Pausing halfway through the cooking time to flip the chicken, air fry for 20 to 25 minutes, until a thermometer inserted into the thickest part registers 165°F (74°C).
6. While the chicken is baking, prepare the sauce. In a small pan over medium heat, simmer the balsamic vinegar until thick and syrupy, about 5 minutes. Set aside until the chicken is done. When ready to serve, warm the sauce over medium heat and whisk in the butter, 1 tablespoon at a time, until melted and smooth. Season to taste with salt and pepper.
7. Serve the chicken breasts with the sauce drizzled on top.

Per Serving

calories: 510 | fat: 32g | protein: 50g | carbs: 7g | net carbs: 7g | fiber: 0g

Bacon Spinach Chicken

Prep time: 15 minutes | Cook time: 20 minutes | Serves 4

3 tablespoons pine nuts

¾ cup frozen spinach, thawed and squeezed dry

⅓ cup ricotta cheese

2 tablespoons grated Parmesan cheese

3 cloves garlic, minced

Salt and freshly ground black pepper

4 small boneless, skinless chicken breast halves (about 1½ pounds / 680g)

8 slices bacon

1. Place the pine nuts in a small pan and set in the air fryer basket. Set the air fryer to 400°F (205°C) and air fry for 2 to 3 minutes until toasted. Remove the pine nuts to a mixing bowl and continue preheating the air fryer.
2. In a large bowl, combine the spinach, ricotta, Parmesan, and garlic. Season to taste with salt and pepper and stir well until thoroughly combined.

3. Using a sharp knife, cut into the chicken breasts, slicing them across and opening them up like a book, but be careful not to cut them all the way through. Sprinkle the chicken with salt and pepper.
4. Spoon equal amounts of the spinach mixture into the chicken, then fold the top of the chicken breast back over the top of the stuffing. Wrap each chicken breast with 2 slices of bacon.
5. Working in batches if necessary, air fry the chicken for 18 to 20 minutes until the bacon is crisp and a thermometer inserted into the thickest part of the chicken registers 165°F (74°C).

Per Serving

calories: 440 | fat: 20g | protein: 63g | carbs: 4g | net carbs: 3g | fiber: 1g

Broccoli Cheese Chicken

Prep time: 10 minutes | Cook time: 19 to 24 minutes | Serves 6

1 tablespoon avocado oil

¼ cup chopped onion

½ cup finely chopped broccoli

4 ounces (113 g) cream cheese, at room temperature

2 ounces (57 g) Cheddar cheese, shredded

1 teaspoon garlic powder

½ teaspoon sea salt, plus additional for seasoning, divided

¼ freshly ground black pepper, plus additional for seasoning, divided

2 pounds (907 g) boneless, skinless chicken breasts

1 teaspoon smoked paprika

1. Heat a medium skillet over medium-high heat and pour in the avocado oil. Add the onion and broccoli and cook, stirring occasionally, for 5 to 8 minutes, until the onion is tender.
2. Transfer to a large bowl and stir in the cream cheese, Cheddar cheese, and garlic powder, and season to taste with salt and pepper.
3. Hold a sharp knife parallel to the chicken breast and cut a long pocket into one side. Stuff the chicken pockets with the broccoli mixture, using toothpicks to secure the pockets around the filling.
4. In a small dish, combine the paprika, ½ teaspoon salt, and ¼ teaspoon pepper. Sprinkle this over the outside of the chicken.

5. Set the air fryer to 400°F (205ºC). Place the chicken in a single layer in the air fryer basket, cooking in batches if necessary, and cook for 14 to 16 minutes, until an instant-read thermometer reads 160°F (71ºC). Place the chicken on a plate and tent a piece of aluminum foil over the chicken. Allow to rest for 5 to 10 minutes before serving.

Per Serving

calories: 277 | fat: 15g | protein: 35g | carbs: 3g | net carbs: 2g | fiber: 1g

Chicken Broccoli Casserole with Cheese

Prep time: 15 minutes | Cook time: 25 minutes | Serves 4

½ pound (227g) broccoli, chopped into florets

2 cups shredded cooked chicken

4 ounces (113 g) cream cheese

⅓ cup heavy cream

1½ teaspoons Dijon mustard

½ teaspoon garlic powder

Salt and freshly ground black pepper

2 tablespoons chopped fresh basil

1 cup shredded Cheddar cheese

1. Preheat the air fryer to 390°F (199ºC). Lightly coat a 6-cup casserole dish that will fit in air fryer, such an 8-inch round pan, with olive oil and set aside.
2. Place the broccoli in a large glass bowl with 1 tablespoon of water and cover with a microwavable plate. Microwave on high for 2 to 3 minutes until the broccoli is bright green but not mushy. Drain if necessary and add to another large bowl along with the shredded chicken.
3. In the same glass bowl used to microwave the broccoli, combine the cream cheese and cream. Microwave for 30 seconds to 1 minute on high and stir until smooth. Add the mustard and garlic powder and season to taste with salt and freshly ground black pepper. Whisk until the sauce is smooth.
4. Pour the warm sauce over the broccoli and chicken mixture and then add the basil. Using a silicone spatula, gently fold the mixture until thoroughly combined.
5. Transfer the chicken mixture to the prepared casserole dish and top with the cheese. Air fry for 20 to 25 minutes until warmed through and the cheese has browned.

Per Serving

calories: 430 | fat: 32g | protein: 29g | carbs: 6g | net carbs: 5g | fiber: 1g

Chicken Croquettes with Creole Sauce

Prep time: 10 minutes | Cook time: 10 minutes | Serves 4

2 cups shredded cooked chicken
½ cup shredded Cheddar cheese
2 eggs
¼ cup finely chopped onion
¼ cup almond meal
1 tablespoon poultry seasoning
Olive oil

Creole Sauce:
¼ cup mayonnaise
¼ cup sour cream
1½ teaspoons Dijon mustard
1½ teaspoons fresh lemon juice
½ teaspoon garlic powder
½ teaspoon Creole seasoning

1. In a large bowl, combine the chicken, Cheddar, eggs, onion, almond meal, and poultry seasoning. Stir gently until thoroughly combined. Cover and refrigerate for 30 minutes.
2. Meanwhile, to make the Creole sauce: In a small bowl, whisk together the mayonnaise, sour cream, Dijon mustard, lemon juice, garlic powder, and Creole seasoning until thoroughly combined. Cover and refrigerate until ready to serve.
3. Preheat the air fryer to 400°F (205°C). Divide the chicken mixture into 8 portions and shape into patties.
4. Working in batches if necessary, arrange the patties in a single layer in the air fryer basket and coat both sides lightly with olive oil. Pausing halfway through the cooking time to flip the patties, air fry for 10 minutes, or until lightly browned and the cheese is melted. Serve with the Creole sauce.

Per Serving

calories: 380 | fat: 28g | protein: 29g | carbs: 4g | net carbs: 4g | fiber: 0g

Aromatic Chicken Thigh

Prep time: 10 minutes | Cook time: 20 minutes | Serves 6

¼ cup plain Greek yogurt

2 cloves garlic, minced

1 tablespoon grated fresh ginger

½ teaspoon ground cayenne

½ teaspoon ground turmeric

½ teaspoon garam masala

1 teaspoon ground cumin

1 teaspoon salt

2 pounds (907 g) boneless chicken thighs, skin on

2 tablespoons chopped fresh cilantro

1 lemon, cut into 6 wedges

½ sweet onion, sliced

1. In a small bowl, combine the yogurt, garlic, ginger, cayenne, turmeric, garam masala, cumin, and salt. Whisk until thoroughly combined.
2. Transfer the yogurt mixture to a large resealable bag. Add the chicken, seal the bag, and massage the bag to ensure chicken is evenly coated. Refrigerate for 1 hour (or up to 8 hours).
3. Preheat the air fryer to 360°F (182°C).
4. Remove the chicken from the marinade (discard the marinade) and arrange in a single layer in the air fryer basket. Pausing halfway through the cooking time to flip the chicken, air fry for 15 to 20 minutes, until a thermometer inserted into the thickest part registers 165°F (74°C).
5. Transfer the chicken to a serving platter. Top with the cilantro and serve with the lemon wedges and sliced onion.

Per Serving

calories: 350 | fat: 22g | protein: 35g | carbs: 1g | net carbs: 1g | fiber: 0g

Ham Chicken with Cheese

Prep time: 15 minutes | Cook time: 25 minutes | Serves 4

¼ cup unsalted butter, softened

4 ounces (113 g) cream cheese, softened

1½ teaspoons Dijon mustard

2 tablespoons white wine vinegar

¼ cup water

2 cups shredded cooked chicken

¼ pound (113 g) ham, chopped

4 ounces (113 g) sliced Swiss or Provolone cheese

1. Preheat the air fryer to 380°F (193ºC). Lightly coat a 6-cup casserole dish that will fit in the air fryer, such as an 8-inch round pan, with olive oil and set aside.
2. In a large bowl and using an electric mixer, combine the butter, cream cheese, Dijon mustard, and vinegar. With the motor running on low speed, slowly add the water and beat until smooth. Set aside.
3. Arrange an even layer of chicken in the bottom of the prepared pan, followed by the ham. Spread the butter and cream cheese mixture on top of the ham, followed by the cheese slices on the top layer. Air fry for 20 to 25 minutes until warmed through and the cheese has browned.

Per Serving

calories: 480 | fat: 36g | protein: 34g | carbs: 4g | net carbs: 4g | fiber: 0g

Cheey Chicken with Sauce

Prep time: 15 minutes | Cook time: 20 minutes | Serves 4

2 large skinless chicken breasts (about 1¼ pounds / 567g)

Salt and freshly ground black pepper

½ cup almond meal

½ cup grated Parmesan cheese

2 teaspoons Italian seasoning

1 egg, lightly beaten

1 tablespoon olive oil

1 cup no-sugar-added marinara sauce

4 slices Mozzarella cheese or ½ cup shredded Mozzarella

1. Preheat the air fryer to 360°F (182ºC).

2. Slice the chicken breasts in half horizontally to create 4 thinner chicken breasts. Working with one piece at a time, place the chicken between two pieces of parchment paper and pound with a meat mallet or rolling pin to flatten to an even thickness. Season both sides with salt and freshly ground black pepper.
3. In a large shallow bowl, combine the almond meal, Parmesan, and Italian seasoning; stir until thoroughly combined. Place the egg in another large shallow bowl.
4. Dip the chicken in the egg, followed by the almond meal mixture, pressing the mixture firmly into the chicken to create an even coating.
5. Working in batches if necessary, arrange the chicken breasts in a single layer in the air fryer basket and coat both sides lightly with olive oil. Pausing halfway through the cooking time to flip the chicken, air fry for 15 minutes, or until a thermometer inserted into the thickest part registers 165°F (74°C).
6. Spoon the marinara sauce over each piece of chicken and top with the Mozzarella cheese. Air fry for an additional 3 to 5 minutes until the cheese is melted.

Per Serving

calories: 460 | fat: 16g | protein: 65g | carbs: 11g | net carbs: 9g | fiber: 2g

Buttery Chicken

Prep time:25 minutes | Cook time: 14 to 18 minutes | Serves 8

½ cup (1 stick) unsalted butter, at room temperature

1 teaspoon minced garlic

2 tablespoons chopped fresh parsley

½ teaspoon freshly ground black pepper

2 pounds (907 g) boneless, skinless chicken breasts

Sea salt

¾ cup finely ground blanched almond flour

¾ cup grated Parmesan cheese

⅛ teaspoon cayenne pepper

2 large eggs

Avocado oil spray

1. In a medium bowl, combine the butter, garlic, parsley, and black pepper. Form the mixture into a log and wrap it tightly with parchment paper or plastic wrap. Refrigerate for at least 2 hours, until firm.

2. Place the chicken breasts in a zip-top bag or between two pieces of plastic wrap. Pound the chicken with a meat mallet or heavy skillet to an even ¼-inch thickness.
3. Place a pat of butter in the center of each chicken breast and wrap the chicken tightly around the butter from the long side, tucking in the short sides as you go. Secure with toothpicks. Season the outside of the chicken with salt. Wrap the stuffed chicken tightly with plastic wrap and refrigerate at least 2 hours or overnight.
4. In a shallow bowl, combine the almond flour, Parmesan cheese, and cayenne pepper.
5. In another shallow bowl, beat the eggs.
6. Dip each piece of chicken in the eggs, then coat it in the almond flour mixture, using your fingers to press the breading gently into the chicken.
7. Set the air fryer to 350°F (180ºC). Spray the chicken with oil and place it in a single layer in the air fryer basket, working in batches if necessary. Cook for 8 minutes. Flip the chicken, then spray it again with oil. Cook for 6 to 10 minutes more, until an instant-read thermometer reads 165°F (74ºC).

Per Serving

calories: 333 | fat: 23g | protein: 31g | carbs: 3g | net carbs: 2g | fiber: 1g

Air Fried Chicken

Prep time: 20 minutes | Cook time: 7 to 10 minutes | Serves 4

1 pound (454 g) boneless, skinless chicken breasts or thighs

2 tablespoons avocado oil

1 tablespoon freshly squeezed lemon juice

1 teaspoon chopped fresh oregano

½ teaspoon garlic powder

Sea salt

Freshly ground black pepper

1. Place the chicken in a zip-top bag or between two pieces of plastic wrap. Using a meat mallet or a heavy skillet, pound the chicken until it is very thin, about ¼-inch thick.
2. In a small bowl, combine the avocado oil, lemon juice, oregano, garlic powder, salt, and pepper. Place the chicken in a shallow dish and pour the marinade over it. Toss to coat all the chicken, and let it rest at room temperature for 10 to 15 minutes.
3. Set the air fryer to 400°F (205ºC). Place the chicken in a single layer in the air fryer basket and cook for 5 minutes. Flip and cook for another 2 to 5 minutes, until an instant-read thermometer reads 160°F (71ºC). Allow to rest for 5 minutes before serving.

Per Serving

calories: 178 | fat: 10g | protein: 23g | carbs: 2g | net carbs: 1g | fiber: 1g

Spicy Cheese Chicken Roll-Up

Prep time: 10 minutes | Cook time: 14 to 17 minutes | Serves 8

2 pounds (907 g) boneless, skinless chicken breasts or thighs

1 teaspoon chili powder

½ teaspoon smoked paprika

½ teaspoon ground cumin

Sea salt

Freshly ground black pepper

6 ounces (170 g) Monterey Jack cheese, shredded

4 ounces (113 g) canned diced green chiles

Avocado oil spray

1. Place the chicken in a large zip-top bag or between two pieces of plastic wrap. Using a meat mallet or heavy skillet, pound the chicken until it is about ¼ -inch thick.
2. In a small bowl, combine the chili powder, smoked paprika, cumin, and salt and pepper to taste. Sprinkle both sides of the chicken with the seasonings.
3. Sprinkle the chicken with the Monterey Jack cheese, then the diced green chiles.
4. Roll up each piece of chicken from the long side, tucking in the ends as you go. Secure the roll-up with a toothpick.
5. Set the air fryer to 350°F (180°C). Spray the outside of the chicken with avocado oil. Place the chicken in a single layer in the basket, working in batches if necessary, and cook for 7 minutes. Flip and cook for another 7 to 10 minutes, until an instant-read thermometer reads 160°F (71°C).
6. Remove the chicken from the air fryer and allow it to rest for about 5 minutes before serving.

Per Serving

calories: 192 | fat: 9g | protein: 28g | carbs: 2g | net carbs: 1g | fiber: 1g

Cheesy Chicken

Prep time: 10 minutes | Cook time: 14 to 17 minutes | Serves 8

2 pounds (907 g) boneless, skinless chicken breasts or thighs

Sea salt

Freshly ground black pepper

8 ounces (227 g) cream cheese, at room temperature

4 ounces (113 g) Cheddar cheese, shredded

2 jalapeños, seeded and diced

1 teaspoon minced garlic

Avocado oil spray

1. Place the chicken in a large zip-top bag or between two pieces of plastic wrap. Using a meat mallet or heavy skillet, pound the chicken until it is about ¼-inch thick. Season both sides of the chicken with salt and pepper.
2. In a medium bowl, combine the cream cheese, Cheddar cheese, jalapeños, and garlic. Divide the mixture among the chicken pieces. Roll up each piece from the long side, tucking in the ends as you go. Secure with toothpicks.
3. Set the air fryer to 350°F (180°C). Spray the outside of the chicken with oil. Place the chicken in a single layer in the air fryer basket, working in batches if necessary, and cook for 7 minutes. Flip the chicken and cook for another 7 to 10 minutes, until an instant-read thermometer reads 160°F (71°C).

Per Serving

calories: 264 | fat: 17g | protein: 28g | carbs: 2g | net carbs: 1g | fiber: 1g

Aromatic Chicken Leg

Prep time: 5 minutes | Cook time: 23 to 27 minutes | Serves 6

½ cup avocado oil

2 teaspoons smoked paprika

1 teaspoon sea salt

1 teaspoon garlic powder

½ teaspoon dried rosemary

½ teaspoon dried thyme

½ teaspoon freshly ground black pepper

2 pounds (907 g) bone-in, skin-on chicken leg quarters

1. In a blender or small bowl, combine the avocado oil, smoked paprika, salt, garlic powder, rosemary, thyme, and black pepper.
2. Place the chicken in a shallow dish or large zip-top bag. Pour the marinade over the chicken, making sure all the legs are coated. Cover and marinate for at least 2 hours or overnight.
3. Place the chicken in a single layer in the air fryer basket, working in batches if necessary. Set the air fryer to 400°F (205ºC) and cook for 15 minutes. Flip the chicken legs, then reduce the temperature to 350°F (180ºC). Cook for 8 to 12 minutes more, until an instant-read thermometer reads 160°F (71ºC) when inserted into the thickest piece of chicken.
4. Allow to rest for 5 to 10 minutes before serving.

Per Serving

calories: 569 | fat: 53g | protein: 23g | carbs: 2g | net carbs: 1g | fiber: 1g

Chicken Legs with Turnip

Prep time: 30 minutes | Cook time: 25 minutes | Serves 3

1 pound (454 g) chicken legs

1 teaspoon Himalayan salt

1 teaspoon paprika

½ teaspoon ground black pepper

1 teaspoon butter, melted

1 turnip, trimmed and sliced

1. Spritz the sides and bottom of the cooking basket with a nonstick cooking spray.
2. Season the chicken legs with salt, paprika, and ground black pepper.
3. Cook at 370 degrees F (188ºC) for 10 minutes. Increase the temperature to 380 degrees F (193ºC).
4. Drizzle turnip slices with melted butter and transfer them to the cooking basket with the chicken. Cook the turnips and chicken for 15 minutes more, flipping them halfway through the cooking time.
5. As for the chicken, an instant-read thermometer should read at least 165 degrees F (74ºC).
6. Serve and enjoy!

Per Serving

calories: 207 | fat: 7g | protein: 29g | carbs: 3g | net carbs: 2g | fiber: 1g

Chicken with Brussels Sprouts

Prep time: 30 minutes | Cook time: 35 minutes | Serves 2

2 chicken legs

½ teaspoon paprika

½ teaspoon kosher salt

½ teaspoon black pepper

½ pound (227g) Brussels sprouts

1 teaspoon dill, fresh or dried

1. Start by preheating your Air Fryer to 370 degrees F (188ºC).
2. Now, season your chicken with paprika, salt, and pepper. Transfer the chicken legs to the cooking basket. Cook for 10 minutes.
3. Flip the chicken legs and cook an additional 10 minutes. Reserve.
4. Add the Brussels sprouts to the cooking basket; sprinkle with dill. Cook at 380 degrees F (193ºC) for 15 minutes, shaking the basket halfway through.
5. Serve with the reserved chicken legs. Bon appétit!

Per Serving

calories: 365 | fat: 20g | protein: 14g | carbs: 25g | net carbs: 21g | fiber: 4g

Roast Chicken Leg

Prep time: 20 minutes | Cook time: 18 minutes | Serves 6

2 leeks, sliced

2 large-sized tomatoes, chopped

3 cloves garlic, minced

½ teaspoon dried oregano

6 chicken legs, boneless and skinless

½ teaspoon smoked cayenne pepper

2 tablespoons olive oil

A freshly ground nutmeg

1. In a mixing dish, thoroughly combine all ingredients, minus the leeks. Place in the refrigerator and let it marinate overnight.
2. Lay the leeks onto the bottom of an Air Fryer cooking basket. Top with the chicken legs.
3. Roast chicken legs at 375 degrees F (190ºC) for 18 minutes, turning halfway through. Serve with hoisin sauce.

Per Serving

calories: 390 | fat: 15g | protein: 12g | carbs: 7g | net carbs: 6g | fiber: 1g

Cheesy Sausage Zucchini Casserole

Prep time: 50 minutes | Cook time: 16 minutes | Serves 4

8 ounces (227 g) zucchini, spiralized

1 pound (454 g) smoked chicken sausage, sliced

1 tomato, puréed

½ cup Asiago cheese, shredded

1 tablespoon Italian seasoning mix

3 tablespoons Romano cheese, grated

1 tablespoon fresh basil leaves, chiffonade

1. Salt the zucchini and let it stand for 30 minutes; pat it dry with kitchen towels.
2. Then, spritz a baking pan with cooking spray; add the zucchini to the pan. Stir in the chicken sausage, tomato purée, Asiago cheese, and Italian seasoning mix.
3. Bake in the preheated Air Fryer at 325 degrees F (163ºC) for 11 minutes.
4. Top with the grated Romano cheese. Turn the temperature to 390 degrees F (199ºC) and cook an additional 5 minutes or until everything is thoroughly heated and the cheese is melted.
5. Garnish with fresh basil leaves. Bon appétit!

Per Serving

calories: 300 | fat: 17g | protein: 5g | carbs: 9g | net carbs: 7g | fiber: 2g

Air Fried Chicken Drumettes

Prep time: 15 minutes | Cook time: 22 minutes | Serves 3

1/3 cup almond meal

½ teaspoon ground white pepper

1 teaspoon seasoning salt

1 teaspoon garlic paste

1 teaspoon rosemary

1 whole egg + 1 egg white

6 chicken drumettes

1 heaping tablespoon fresh chives, chopped

1. Start by preheating your Air Fryer to 390 degrees (199ºC).
2. Mix the almond meal with white pepper, salt, garlic paste, and rosemary in a small-sized bowl.
3. In another bowl, beat the eggs until frothy.
4. Dip the chicken into the flour mixture, then into the beaten eggs; coat with the flour mixture one more time.
5. Cook the chicken drumettes for 22 minutes. Serve warm, garnished with chives.

Per Serving

calories: 319 | fat: 11g | protein: 4g | carbs: 22g | net carbs: 21g | fiber: 1g

Chicken Wing with Piri Piri Sauce

Prep time: 1 hour 30 minutes | Cook time: 30 minutes | Serves 6

12 chicken wings

1½ ounces (43 g) butter, melted

1 teaspoon onion powder

½ teaspoon cumin powder

1 teaspoon garlic paste

For the Sauce:

2 ounces (57 g) piri piri peppers, stemmed and chopped

1 tablespoon pimiento, seeded and minced

1 garlic clove, chopped

2 tablespoons fresh lemon juice

⅓ teaspoon sea salt

½ teaspoon tarragon

1. Steam the chicken wings using a steamer basket that is placed over a saucepan with boiling water; reduce the heat.
2. Now, steam the wings for 10 minutes over a moderate heat. Toss the wings with butter, onion powder, cumin powder, and garlic paste.
3. Let the chicken wings cool to room temperature. Then, refrigerate them for 45 to 50 minutes.
4. Roast in the preheated Air Fryer at 330 degrees F (166ºC) for 25 to 30 minutes; make sure to flip them halfway through.
5. While the chicken wings are cooking, prepare the sauce by mixing all of the sauce ingredients in a food processor. Toss the wings with prepared Piri Piri Sauce and serve.

Per Serving

calories: 517 | fat: 21g | protein: 4g | carbs: 12g | net carbs: 11g | fiber: 1g

Creamy Chicken

Prep time: 20 minutes | Cook time: 18 minutes | Serves 4

½ cup full-fat sour cream

1 teaspoon ground cinnamon

½ teaspoon whole grain mustard

1½ tablespoons mayonnaise

1 pound (454 g) chicken thighs, boneless, skinless, and cut into pieces

1½ tablespoons olive oil

2 heaping tablespoons fresh rosemary, minced

½ cup white wine

3 cloves garlic, minced

½ teaspoon smoked paprika

Salt and freshly cracked black pepper, to taste

1. Firstly, in a mixing dish, combine chicken thighs with olive oil and white wine; stir to coat.
2. After that, throw in the garlic, smoked paprika, ground cinnamon, salt, and black pepper; cover and refrigerate for 1 to 3 hours.

3. Set the Air Fryer to cook at 375 degrees F (190ºC). Roast the chicken thighs for 18 minutes, turning halfway through and working in batches.
4. To make the sauce, combine the sour cream, whole grain mustard, mayonnaise and rosemary. Serve the turkey with the mustard/rosemary sauce and enjoy!

Per Serving

calories: 362 | fat: 27g | protein: 8g | carbs: 17g | net carbs: 16g | fiber: 1g

Cheese Chicken Burgers

Prep time: 10 minutes | Cook time: 15 minutes | Serves 4

1 palmful dried basil

1/3 cup Parmesan cheese, grated

2 teaspoons dried marjoram

1/3 teaspoon ancho chili powder

2 teaspoons dried parsley flakes

½ teaspoon onion powder

Toppings, to serve

1/3 teaspoon porcini powder

1 teaspoon sea salt flakes

1 pound (454 g) chicken meat, ground

2 teaspoons cumin powder

1/3 teaspoon red pepper flakes, crushed

1 teaspoon freshly cracked black pepper

:

1. Generously grease an Air Fryer cooking basket with a thin layer of olive oil.
2. In a mixing dish, combine chicken meat with all seasonings. Shape into 4 patties and coat them with grated Parmesan cheese.
3. Cook chicken burgers in the preheated Air Fryer for 15 minutes at 345 degrees F (174ºC), working in batches, flipping them once.
4. Serve with toppings of choice. Bon appétit!

Per Serving

calories: 234 | fat: 12g | protein: 6g | carbs: 12g | net carbs: 11g | fiber: 1g

Aromatic Chicken with Cauliflower

Prep time: 15 minutes | Cook time: 28 minutes | Serves 6

2 handful fresh Italian parsleys, roughly chopped

½ cup fresh chopped chives

2 sprigs thyme

6 chicken drumsticks

1½ small-sized head cauliflower, broken into large-sized florets

2 teaspoons mustard powder

$^1/_3$ teaspoon porcini powder

1 ½ teaspoons berbere spice

$^1/_3$ teaspoon sweet paprika

½ teaspoon shallot powder

1 teaspoon granulated garlic

1 teaspoon freshly cracked pink peppercorns

½ teaspoon sea salt

1. Simply combine all items for the berbere spice rub mix. After that, coat the chicken drumsticks with this rub mix on all sides. Transfer them to the baking dish.
2. Now, lower the cauliflower onto the chicken drumsticks. Add thyme, chives and Italian parsley and spritz everything with a pan spray. Transfer the baking dish to the preheated Air Fryer.
3. Next step, set the timer for 28 minutes; roast at 355 degrees F (181ºC), turning occasionally. Bon appétit!

Per Serving

calories: 350 | fat: 12g | protein: 18g | carbs: 13g | net carbs: 11g | fiber: 2g

White Wine Chicken Breast

Prep time: 30 minutes | Cook time: 28 minutes | Serves 4

½ teaspoon grated fresh ginger

$1/3$ cup coconut milk

½ teaspoon sea salt flakes

3 medium-sized boneless chicken breasts, cut into small pieces

1½ tablespoons sesame oil

3 green garlic stalks, finely chopped

½ cup dry white wine

½ teaspoon fresh thyme leaves, minced

$1/3$ teaspoon freshly cracked black pepper

:

1. Warm the sesame oil in a deep sauté pan over a moderate heat. Then, sauté the green garlic until just fragrant.
2. Remove the pan from the heat and pour in the coconut milk and the white wine. After that, add the thyme, sea salt, fresh ginger, and freshly cracked black pepper. Scrape this mixture into a baking dish.
3. Stir in the chicken chunks.
4. Cook in the preheated Air Fryer for 28 minutes at 335 degrees F (168ºC). Serve on individual plates and eat warm.

Per Serving

calories: 471 | fat: 28g | protein: 12g | carbs: 31g | net carbs: 31g | fiber: 0g

Air Fried Cheesy Chicken

Prep time: 10 minutes | Cook time: 10 minutes | Serves 4

2 ounces (57 g) Asiago cheese, cut into sticks

$1/3$ cup keto tomato paste

½ teaspoon garlic paste

2 chicken breasts, cut in half lengthwise

½ cup green onions, chopped

1 tablespoon chili sauce

½ cup roasted vegetable stock

1 tablespoon sesame oil

1 teaspoon salt

2 teaspoons unsweetened cocoa

½ teaspoon sweet paprika, or more to taste

1. Sprinkle chicken breasts with the salt and sweet paprika; drizzle with chili sauce. Now, place a stick of Asiago cheese in the middle of each chicken breast.
2. Then, tie the whole thing using a kitchen string; give a drizzle of sesame oil.
3. Transfer the stuffed chicken to the cooking basket. Add the other ingredients and toss to coat the chicken.
4. Afterward, cook for about 11 minutes at 395 degrees F (202ºC). Serve the chicken on two serving plates, garnish with fresh or pickled salad and serve immediately. Bon appétit!

Per Serving

calories: 390 | fat: 12g | protein: 2g | carbs: 8g | net carbs: 7g | fiber: 1g

Chicken Vegetable with Cheese

Prep time: 25 minutes | Cook time: 22 minutes | Serves 4

3 eggs, whisked

½ teaspoon dried marjoram

$1/3$ cup Fontina cheese, grated

1 teaspoon sea salt

$1/3$ teaspoon red pepper flakes, crushed

2 cups leftover keto vegetables

½ red onion, thinly sliced

2 cups cooked chicken, shredded or chopped

3 cloves garlic, finely minced

1. Simply mix all of the above ingredients, except for cheese, with a wide spatula.
2. Scrape the mixture into a previously greased baking dish.
3. Set your Air Fryer to cook at 365 degrees F (185ºC) for 22 minutes. Air-fry until everything is bubbling. Serve warm topped with grated Fontina cheese. Bon appétit!

Per Serving

calories: 361 | fat: 29g | protein: 1g | carbs: 24g | net carbs: 23g | fiber: 1g

Cheesy Chicken with Bacon

Prep time: 10 minutes | Cook time: 13 minutes | Serves 2

4 rashers smoked bacon

2 chicken fillets

½ teaspoon coarse sea salt

¼ teaspoon black pepper, preferably freshly ground

1 teaspoon garlic, minced

1 (2-inch) piece ginger, peeled and minced

1 teaspoon black mustard seeds

1 teaspoon mild curry powder

½ cup coconut milk

½ cup Parmesan cheese, grated

1. Start by preheating your Air Fryer to 400 degrees F (205ºC). Add the smoked bacon and cook in the preheated Air Fryer for 5 to 7 minutes. Reserve.
2. In a mixing bowl, place the chicken fillets, salt, black pepper, garlic, ginger, mustard seeds, curry powder, and milk. Let it marinate in your refrigerator about 30 minutes.
3. In another bowl, place the grated Parmesan cheese.
4. Dredge the chicken fillets through the Parmesan mixture and transfer them to the cooking basket. Reduce the temperature to 380 degrees F (193ºC) and cook the chicken for 6 minutes.
5. Turn them over and cook for a further 6 minutes. Repeat the process until you have run out of ingredients.
6. Serve with reserved bacon. Enjoy!

Per Serving

calories: 612 | fat: 44g | protein: 16g | carbs: 38g | net carbs: 37g | fiber: 1g

Chicken with Bacon and Tomato

Prep time: 25 minutes | Cook time: 10 minutes | Serves 4

4 medium-sized skin-on chicken drumsticks

1½ teaspoons herbs de Provence

Salt and pepper, to taste

1 tablespoon rice vinegar

2 tablespoons olive oil

2 garlic cloves, crushed

12 ounces (340 g) crushed canned tomatoes

1 small-size leek, thinly sliced

2 slices smoked bacon, chopped

1. Sprinkle the chicken drumsticks with herbs de Provence, salt and pepper; then, drizzle them with rice vinegar and olive oil.
2. Cook in the baking pan at 360 degrees F (182ºC) for 8 to 10 minutes.
3. Pause the Air Fryer; stir in the remaining ingredients and continue to cook for 15 minutes longer; make sure to check them periodically. Bon appétit!

Per Serving

calories: 296 | fat: 13g | protein: 34g | carbs: 7g | net carbs: 5g | fiber: 2g

Spicy Chicken

Prep time: 20 minutes | Cook time: 18 minutes | Serves 4

$1/3$ teaspoon paprika

$1/3$ cup scallions, peeled and chopped

3 cloves garlic, peeled and minced

1 teaspoon ground black pepper, or to taste

½ teaspoon fresh basil, minced

1½ cups chicken, minced

1½ tablespoons coconut aminos

½ teaspoon grated fresh ginger

½ tablespoon chili sauce

1 teaspoon salt

:

1. Thoroughly combine all ingredients in a mixing dish. Then, form into 4 patties.
2. Cook in the preheated Air Fryer for 18 minutes at 355 degrees F (181ºC).

3. Garnish with toppings of choice. Bon appétit!

Per Serving

calories: 366 | fat: 9g | protein: 11g | carbs: 34g | net carbs: 33g | fiber: 1g

Air Fried Chicken Kebabs

Prep time: 15 minutes | Cook time: 20 minutes | Serves 5

¼ diced red onion

½ diced zucchini

½ diced red pepper

½ diced green pepper

½ diced yellow pepper

1 teaspoon BBQ seasoning

1 tablespoon chicken seasoning

2 tablespoons coconut aminos

5 grape tomatoes

16 ounces (454 g) 1-inch cubed chicken breasts

Salt & pepper, to taste

Nonstick cooking oil spray

1. Pat dry the chicken breasts then combine the BBQ seasoning, chicken seasoning, salt, pepper and coconut aminos together.
2. Generously coat the chicken cubes with the mixture then set aside to marinate for about an hour.
3. Sew the marinated chicken cubes onto the wooden skewers.
4. Alternatively layer the chicken cubes with onions, zucchini, pepper and top each skewer with a grape tomato.
5. Spray the layered skewers with the cooking oil then line the fryer basket with parchment paper and fit in a small grill rack.
6. Place the skewers on the grill rack then air fry at 350°F (180°C) for 10 minutes.
7. Flip the skewers over and fry for an additional 10 minutes.
8. Allow the chicken to cool for a bit then serve and enjoy with any sauce of choice.

Per Serving

calories: 255 | fat: 12g | protein: 25g | carbs: 6g | net carbs: 5g | fiber: 1g

Chicken Nuggets

Prep time: 10 minutes | Cook time: 12 minutes | Serves 4

⅛ teaspoon sea salt

¼ cup coconut flour

½ teaspoon ground ginger

1 teaspoon sesame oil

1-pound (454-g) chicken breast, boneless & skinless

4 large egg whites

6 tablespoons toasted sesame seeds

nonstick cooking oil spray

for the dip

½ teaspoon monk fruit

½ teaspoon ground ginger

1 tablespoon water

1 teaspoon sriracha

2 teaspoons rice vinegar

2 tablespoons almond butter

4 teaspoons coconut aminos

1. Chop the chicken breast into 1-inch nuggets then pat dry and place in a medium sized mixing bowl.
2. Pour in the sesame oil, salt and massage into the chicken nuggets.
3. Pour the ground ginger and coconut flour into a large ziploc bag then add in the coated chicken nuggets and shake around to coat.
4. Transfer the chicken nuggets into a bowl filled with the egg whites and toss around until covered in the whites.
5. Shake off excess white from the nuggets then cover with the sesame seeds.
6. Heat the fryer up 400°F (205°C) for 10 minutes then coat the basket with oil and add in the covered chicken nuggets and fry for 6 minutes.
7. Flip the chicken nuggets over and cook until crispy for 6 extra minutes.
8. In the meantime, combine all the sauce ingredients together until mixed.
9. Serve the fried nuggets along with the sauce and enjoy as desired.

Per Serving

calories: 293 | fat: 14g | protein: 33g | carbs: 8g | net carbs: 6g | fiber: 2g

Aromatic Chicken Thighs

Prep time: 20 minutes | Cook time: 15 minutes | Serves 4

¼ cup full-fat Greek yogurt

½ teaspoon cayenne pepper

½ teaspoon ground cinnamon

½ teaspoon ground black pepper

1 teaspoon kosher salt

1 teaspoon ground cumin

1 tablespoon juiced lime

1 tablespoon avocado oil

1 teaspoon smoked paprika

1 tablespoon keto tomato paste

1 tablespoon minced garlic

1-pound (454 g) chicken thighs, boneless & skinless

1. Using a large mixing bowl, add in the tomato paste, garlic, oil, juiced lime, cumin, salt, black pepper, cinnamon, paprika, cayenne pepper, yogurt and mix until combined.
2. Add the chicken pieces into the mixing bowl and toss until combined, then set aside to marinate for an hour.
3. Arrange the marinated chicken in the fryer basket then cook for 10 minutes at 370°F (188°C).
4. Flip the chicken over and cook for an additional 5 minutes.
5. Serve and enjoy as desired.

Per Serving

calories: 298 | fat: 23g | protein: 20g | carbs: 4g | net carbs: 3g | fiber: 1g

Savory Hen

Prep time: 20 minutes | Cook time: 20 minutes | Serves 4

¼ cup fish sauce

1 teaspoon turmeric

1 tablespoon coconut aminos

1 chopped jalapeño peppers

1 cup chopped cilantro leaves

2 tablespoon stevia

2 teaspoon ground coriander

2 tablespoon lemongrass paste

2 halved whole cornish game hens, with the giblets removed

8 minced garlic cloves

salt & black pepper, to taste

1. Using a high speed blender, add in the turmeric, salt, coriander, pepper, lemongrass paste, sugar, garlic, cilantro, fish sauce and incorporate together.
2. Add in the broiler chicken and toss together until fully coated with the mixture then set aside to marinate for an hour.
3. Transfer the marinated broiler into the fryer basket and air fry for 10 minutes at 400°F (205ºC).
4. Flip the broiler over then cook for an extra 10 minutes.
5. Serve and enjoy as desired.

Per Serving

calories: 222 | fat: 9g | protein: 14g | carbs: 4g | net carbs: 3g | fiber: 1g

Quick Chicken Breast

Prep time: 10 minutes | Cook time: 15 minutes | Serves 4

For the Chicken:

1 teaspoon turmeric

1 diced large onion

1 tablespoon avocado oil

1 teaspoons garam masala

1 teaspoons smoked paprika

1 teaspoons ground fennel seeds

1-pound (454-g) chicken breast, boneless & skinless

2 teaspoons minced ginger

2 teaspoons minced garlic cloves

nonstick cooking oil spray

salt & cayenne pepper, to taste

To Top:

¼ cup chopped cilantro

2 teaspoons juiced lime

1. Make slight piercing all over the chicken breast then set aside.
2. Using a large mixing bowl add in all the remaining ingredients and combine together.
3. Add the pierced chicken breast into the bowl then set aside for an hour to marinate.
4. Transfer the marinated chicken and veggies into the fryer basket then coat with the cooking oil spray.
5. Cook for 15 minutes at 360°F (182°C) then serve and enjoy with a garnish of cilantro topped with the juiced lime.

Per Serving

calories: 305 | fat: 23g | protein: 19g | carbs: 6g | net carbs: 5g | fiber: 1g

Chicken Drumsticks

Prep time: 5 minutes | Cook time: 25 minutes | Serves 4

¼ cup juiced lemon

½ teaspoon cayenne pepper

½ teaspoon coriander seeds

½ teaspoon whole black peppercorns

1 teaspoon turmeric

1 teaspoon kosher salt

1 teaspoon cumin seeds

1 teaspoon parsley, dried

1 teaspoon oregano, dried

1½ pounds (680g) chicken drumsticks

2 tablespoons coconut oil

1. Using a high speed blender, add in the peppercorns, kosher salt, cayenne pepper, coriander seeds, parsley, oregano, cumin, turmeric and blend together until smooth.
2. Transfer the blended spices into a mixing bowl, then add in the oil, juiced lemon and incorporate together.
3. Add in the drumsticks then toss to coat and allow to marinate for an hour.
4. Arrange the drumsticks in the fryer basket with the skin side up and air fry for 15 minutes at 390°F (199°C).

5. Flip the chicken drumstick over then fry for an extra 10 minutes.
6. Serve and enjoy as desired.

Per Serving

calories: 253 | fat: 17g | protein: 20g | carbs: 2g | net carbs: 1g | fiber: 1g

Cheesy Turkey Meatball

Prep time: 10 minutes | Cook time: 10 minutes | Serves 4

1 red bell pepper, seeded and coarsely chopped

2 cloves garlic, coarsely chopped

¼ cup chopped fresh parsley

1½ pounds (680g) 85% lean ground turkey

1 egg, lightly beaten

½ cup grated Parmesan cheese

1 teaspoon salt

½ teaspoon freshly ground black pepper

1. Preheat the air fryer to 400°F (205ºC).
2. In a food processor fitted with a metal blade, combine the bell pepper, garlic, and parsley. Pulse until finely chopped. Transfer the vegetables to a large mixing bowl.
3. Add the turkey, egg, Parmesan, salt, and black pepper. Mix gently until thoroughly combined. Shape the mixture into 1¼-inch meatballs.
4. Working in batches if necessary, arrange the meatballs in a single layer in the air fryer basket; coat lightly with olive oil spray. Pausing halfway through the cooking time to shake the basket, air fry for 7 to 10 minutes, until lightly browned and a thermometer inserted into the center of a meatball registers 165°F (74ºC).

Per Serving

calories: 410 | fat: 27g | protein: 38g | carbs: 4g | net carbs: 3g | fiber: 1g

Air Fried Turkey Breast

Prep time: 5 minutes | Cook time: 45 to 55 minutes | Serves 10

1 tablespoon sea salt

1 teaspoon paprika

1 teaspoon onion powder

1 teaspoon garlic powder

½ teaspoon freshly ground black pepper

4 pounds (1.8 kg) bone-in, skin-on turkey breast

2 tablespoons unsalted butter, melted

1. In a small bowl, combine the salt, paprika, onion powder, garlic powder, and pepper.
2. Sprinkle the seasonings all over the turkey. Brush the turkey with some of the melted butter.
3. Set the air fryer to 350°F (180ºC). Place the turkey in the air fryer basket, skin-side down, and cook for 25 minutes.
4. Flip the turkey and brush it with the remaining butter. Continue cooking for another 20 to 30 minutes, until an instant-read thermometer reads 160°F.
5. Remove the turkey breast from the air fryer. Tent a piece of aluminum foil over the turkey, and allow it to rest for about 5 minutes before serving.

Per Serving

calories: 278 | fat: 14g | protein: 34g | carbs: 2g | net carbs: 1g | fiber: 1g

Turkey with Mustard Sauce

Prep time: 13 minutes | Cook time: 18 minutes | Serves 4

½ teaspoon cumin powder

2 pounds (907 g) turkey breasts, quartered

2 cloves garlic, smashed

½ teaspoon hot paprika

2 tablespoons melted butter

1 teaspoon fine sea salt

Freshly cracked mixed peppercorns, to taste

Fresh juice of 1 lemon

For the Mustard Sauce:

1½ tablespoons mayonnaise

1½ cups Greek yogurt

½ tablespoon yellow mustard

1. Grab a medium-sized mixing dish and combine together the garlic and melted butter; rub this mixture evenly over the surface of the turkey.
2. Add the cumin powder, followed by paprika, salt, peppercorns, and lemon juice. Place in your refrigerator at least 55 minutes.
3. Set your Air Fryer to cook at 375 degrees F (190ºC). Roast the turkey for 18 minutes, turning halfway through; roast in batches.
4. In the meantime, make the mustard sauce by mixing all ingredients for the sauce. Serve warm roasted turkey with the mustard sauce. Bon appétit!

Per Serving

calories: 471 | fat: 23g | protein: 16g | carbs: 34g | net carbs: 33g | fiber: 1g

Turkey Breasts with Mustard

Prep time: 1 hour | Cook time: 53 minutes | Serves 4

½ teaspoon dried thyme

1½ pounds (680g) turkey breasts

½ teaspoon dried sage

3 whole star anise

1½ tablespoons olive oil

1½ tablespoons hot mustard

1 teaspoon smoked cayenne pepper

1 teaspoon fine sea salt

1. Set your Air Fryer to cook at 365 degrees F (185ºC).
2. Brush the turkey breast with olive oil and sprinkle with seasonings.
3. Cook at 365 degrees F (185ºC) for 45 minutes, turning twice. Now, pause the machine and spread the cooked breast with the hot mustard.
4. Air-fry for 6 to 8 more minutes. Let it rest before slicing and serving. Bon appétit!

Per Serving

calories: 321 | fat: 17g | protein: 3g | carbs: 21g | net carbs: 20g | fiber: 1g

Air Fried Turkey

Prep time: 1 hour | Cook time: 58 minutes | Serves 4

2 tablespoons olive oil

2 pounds (907 g) turkey breasts, bone-in skin-on

Coarse sea salt and ground black pepper, to taste

1 teaspoon fresh basil leaves, chopped

2 tablespoons lemon zest, grated

1. Rub olive oil on all sides of the turkey breasts; sprinkle with salt, pepper, basil, and lemon zest.
2. Place the turkey breasts skin side up on a parchment-lined cooking basket.
3. Cook in the preheated Air Fryer at 330 degrees F (166ºC) for 30 minutes. Now, turn them over and cook an additional 28 minutes.
4. Serve with lemon wedges, if desired. Bon appétit!

Per Serving

calories: 416 | fat: 22g | protein: 49g | carbs: 0g | net carbs: 0g | fiber: 0g

Roast Turkey

Prep time: 50 minutes | Cook time: 45 minutes | Serves 6

2½ pounds (1.1kg) turkey breasts

1 tablespoon fresh rosemary, chopped

1 teaspoon sea salt

½ teaspoon ground black pepper

1 onion, chopped

1 celery stalk, chopped

1. Start by preheating your Air Fryer to 360 degrees F (182ºC). Spritz the sides and bottom of the cooking basket with a nonstick cooking spray.
2. Place the turkey in the cooking basket. Add the rosemary, salt, and black pepper. Cook for 30 minutes in the preheated Air Fryer.
3. Add the onion and celery and cook an additional 15 minutes. Bon appétit!

Per Serving

calories: 316 | fat: 14g | protein: 41g | carbs: 2g | net carbs: 1g | fiber: 1g

Turkey with Gravy

Prep time: 50 minutes | Cook time: 20 minutes | Serves 6

2 teaspoons butter, softened

1 teaspoon dried sage

2 sprigs rosemary, chopped

1 teaspoon salt

¼ teaspoon freshly ground black pepper, or more to taste

1 whole turkey breast

2 tablespoons turkey broth

2 tablespoons whole-grain mustard

1 tablespoon butter

1. Start by preheating your Air Fryer to 360 degrees F (182ºC).
2. To make the rub, combine 2 tablespoons of butter, sage, rosemary, salt, and pepper; mix well to combine and spread it evenly over the surface of the turkey breast.
3. Roast for 20 minutes in an Air Fryer cooking basket. Flip the turkey breast over and cook for a further 15 to 16 minutes. Now, flip it back over and roast for 12 minutes more.
4. While the turkey is roasting, whisk the other ingredients in a saucepan. After that, spread the gravy all over the turkey breast.
5. Let the turkey rest for a few minutes before carving. Bon appétit!

Per Serving

calories: 384 | fat: 8g | protein: 131g | carbs: 2g | net carbs: 1g | fiber: 1g

Air Fried Turkey and Chicken

Prep time: 40 minutes | Cook time: 36 minutes | Serves 4

½ medium-sized leek, chopped

½ red onion, chopped

2 garlic cloves, minced

1 jalapeño pepper, seeded and minced

1 bell pepper, seeded and chopped

2 tablespoons olive oil

1 pound (454 g) ground turkey, 85% lean 15% fat

2 cups tomato purée

2 cups chicken stock

½ teaspoon black peppercorns

Salt, to taste

1 teaspoon chili powder

1 teaspoon mustard seeds

1 teaspoon ground cumin

1. Start by preheating your Air Fryer to 365 degrees F (185ºC).
2. Place the leeks, onion, garlic and peppers in a baking pan; drizzle olive oil evenly over the top. Cook for 4 to 6 minutes.
3. Add the ground turkey. Cook for 6 minutes more or until the meat is no longer pink.
4. Now, add the tomato purée, 1 cup of chicken stock, black peppercorns, salt, chili powder, mustard seeds, and cumin to the baking pan. Cook for 24 minutes, stirring every 7 to 10 minutes.
5. Bon appétit!

Per Serving

calories: 271 | fat: 15g | protein: 6g | carbs: 11g | net carbs: 10g | fiber: 1g

Easy Turkey Drumsticks

Prep time: 25 minutes | Cook time: 23 minutes | Serves 2

1 tablespoon red curry paste

½ teaspoon cayenne pepper

1½ tablespoons minced ginger

2 turkey drumsticks

¼ cup coconut milk

1 teaspoon kosher salt, or more to taste

$^1/_3$ teaspoon ground pepper, to more to taste

1. First of all, place turkey drumsticks with all ingredients in your refrigerator; let it marinate overnight.
2. Cook turkey drumsticks at 380 degrees F (193ºC) for 23 minutes; make sure to flip them over at half-time. Serve with the salad on the side.

Per Serving

calories: 298 | fat: 16g | protein: 12g | carbs: 25g | net carbs: 22g | fiber: 3g

Cheesy Turkey Kabobs

Prep time: 15 minutes | Cook time: 10 minutes | Serves 8

1 cup Parmesan cheese, grated

1½ cups of water

14 ounces (397 g) ground turkey

2 small eggs, beaten

1 teaspoon ground ginger

2½ tablespoons olive oil

1 cup chopped fresh parsley

2 tablespoons almond meal

¾ teaspoon salt

1 heaping teaspoon fresh rosemary, finely chopped

½ teaspoon ground allspice

1. Mix all of the above ingredients in a bowl. Knead the mixture with your hands.
2. Then, take small portions and gently roll them into balls.
3. Now, preheat your Air Fryer to 380 degrees F (193ºC). Air fry for 8 to 10 minutes in the Air Fryer basket. Serve on a serving platter with skewers and eat with your favorite dipping sauce.

Per Serving

calories: 185 | fat: 13g | protein: 14g | carbs: 3g | net carbs: 2g | fiber: 1g

Bacon-Wrapped Turkey with Cheese

Prep time: 20 minutes | Cook time: 13 minutes | Serves 12

1½ small-sized turkey breast, chop into 12 pieces

12 thin slices Asiago cheese

Paprika, to taste

Fine sea salt and ground black pepper, to taste

12 rashers bacon

1. Lay out the bacon rashers; place 1 slice of Asiago cheese on each bacon piece.
2. Top with turkey, season with paprika, salt, and pepper, and roll them up; secure with a cocktail stick.
3. Air-fry at 365 degrees F (185ºC) for 13 minutes. Bon appétit!

Per Serving

calories: 568 | fat: 34g | protein: 5g | carbs: 30g | net carbs: 29g | fiber: 1g

Turkey with Tabasco Sauce

Prep time: 15 minutes | Cook time: 22 minutes | Serves 6

1½ pounds (680g) ground turkey

6 whole eggs, well beaten

1/3 teaspoon smoked paprika

2 egg whites, beaten

Tabasco sauce, for drizzling

2 tablespoons sesame oil

2 leeks, chopped

3 cloves garlic, finely minced

1 teaspoon ground black pepper

½ teaspoon sea salt

1. Warm the oil in a pan over moderate heat; then, sweat the leeks and garlic until tender; stir periodically.
2. Next, grease 6 oven safe ramekins with pan spray. Divide the sautéed mixture among six ramekins.
3. In a bowl, beat the eggs and egg whites using a wire whisk. Stir in the smoked paprika, salt and black pepper; whisk until everything is thoroughly combined. Divide the egg mixture among the ramekins.

4. Air-fry approximately 22 minutes at 345 degrees F (174ºC). Drizzle Tabasco sauce over each portion and serve.

Per Serving

calories: 298 | fat: 15g | protein: 6g | carbs: 25g | net carbs: 24g | fiber: 1g

Turkey Sausage with Cauliflower

Prep time: 45 minutes | Cook time: 28 minutes | Serves 4

1 pound (454 g) ground turkey

1 teaspoon garlic pepper

1 teaspoon garlic powder

1/3 teaspoon dried oregano

½ teaspoon salt

1/3 cup onions, chopped

½ head cauliflower, broken into florets

1/3 teaspoon dried basil

½ teaspoon dried thyme, chopped

1. In a mixing bowl, thoroughly combine the ground turkey, garlic pepper, garlic powder, oregano, salt, and onion; stir well to combine. Spritz a nonstick skillet with pan spray; form the mixture into 4 sausages.
2. Then, cook the sausage over medium heat until they are no longer pink, approximately 12 minutes.
3. Arrange the cauliflower florets at the bottom of a baking dish. Sprinkle with thyme and basil; spritz with pan spray. Top with the turkey sausages.
4. Roast for 28 minutes at 375 degrees F (190ºC), turning once halfway through. Eat warm.

Per Serving

calories: 289 | fat: 25g | protein: 11g | carbs: 3g | net carbs: 2g | fiber: 1g

Beef, Pork, and Lamb

Air Fried Flank Steak

Prep time: 5 minutes | Cook time: 8 to 10 minutes | Serves 6

½ cup avocado oil

¼ cup coconut aminos

1 shallot, minced

1 tablespoon minced garlic

2 tablespoons chopped fresh oregano, or 2 teaspoons dried

1½ teaspoons sea salt

1 teaspoon freshly ground black pepper

¼ teaspoon red pepper flakes

2 pounds (907 g) flank steak

1. In a blender, combine the avocado oil, coconut aminos, shallot, garlic, oregano, salt, black pepper, and red pepper flakes. Process until smooth.
2. Place the steak in a zip-top plastic bag or shallow dish with the marinade. Seal the bag or cover the dish and marinate in the refrigerator for at least 2 hours or overnight.
3. Remove the steak from the bag and discard the marinade.
4. Set the air fryer to 400°F (205ºC). Place the steak in the air fryer basket (if needed, cut into sections and work in batches). Cook for 4 to 6 minutes, flip the steak, and cook for another 4 minutes or until the internal temperature reaches 120°F (49ºC) in the thickest part for medium-rare (or as desired).

Per Serving

calories: 304 | fat: 23g | protein: 16g | carbs: 4g | net carbs: 3g | fiber: 1g

Cheesy Flank Steak

Prep time: 10 minutes | Cook time: 14 minutes | Serves 6

1 pound (454 g) flank steak

1 tablespoon avocado oil

½ teaspoon sea salt

½ teaspoon garlic powder

¼ teaspoon freshly ground black pepper

2 ounces (57 g) goat cheese, crumbled

1 cup baby spinach, chopped

1. Place the steak in a large zip-top bag or between two pieces of plastic wrap. Using a meat mallet or heavy-bottomed skillet, pound the steak to an even ¼-inch thickness.
2. Brush both sides of the steak with the avocado oil.
3. Mix the salt, garlic powder, and pepper in a small dish. Sprinkle this mixture over both sides of the steak.
4. Sprinkle the goat cheese over top, and top that with the spinach.
5. Starting at one of the long sides, roll the steak up tightly. Tie the rolled steak with kitchen string at 3-inch intervals.
6. Set the air fryer to 400°F (205ºC). Place the steak roll-up in the air fryer basket. Cook for 7 minutes. Flip the steak and cook for an additional 7 minutes, until an instant-read thermometer reads 120°F (49ºC) for medium-rare (adjust the cooking time for your desired doneness).

Per Serving

calories: 165 | fat: 9g | protein: 18g | carbs: 1g | net carbs: 0g | fiber: 1g

Cheese Steak with Lettuce

Prep time: 15 minutes | Cook time: 8 to 10 minutes | Serves 4

1 pound (454 g) flank steak

1 teaspoon garlic powder

1 teaspoon ground cumin

½ teaspoon sea salt

½ teaspoon freshly ground black pepper

5 ounces (142 g) shredded romaine lettuce

½ cup crumbled feta cheese

½ cup peeled and diced cucumber

$1/3$ cup sliced red onion

¼ cup seeded and diced tomato

2 tablespoons pitted and sliced black olives

Tzatziki Sauce, for serving

1. Pat the steak dry with paper towels. In a small bowl, combine the garlic powder, cumin, salt, and pepper. Sprinkle this mixture all over the steak, and allow the steak to rest at room temperature for 45 minutes.
2. Preheat the air fryer to 400°F (205ºC). Place the steak in the air fryer basket and cook for 4 minutes. Flip the steak and cook 4 to 6 minutes more, until an instant-read thermometer reads 120°F (49ºC) at the thickest point for medium-rare (or as desired). Remove the steak from the air fryer and let it rest for 5 minutes.
3. Divide the romaine among plates. Top with the feta, cucumber, red onion, tomato, and olives.
4. Thinly slice the steak diagonally. Add the steak to the plates and drizzle with tzatziki sauce before serving.

Per Serving

calories: 244 | fat: 12g | protein: 28g | carbs: 5g | net carbs: 4g | fiber: 1g

Zucchini Noodle with Beef Meatball

Prep time: 15 minutes | Cook time: 11 to 13 minutes | Serves 6

1 pound (454 g) ground beef

1½ teaspoons sea salt, plus more for seasoning

1 large egg, beaten

1 teaspoon gelatin

¾ cup Parmesan cheese

2 teaspoons minced garlic

1 teaspoon Italian seasoning

Freshly ground black pepper, to taste

Avocado oil spray

Keto-friendly marinara sauce,, for serving

6 ounces (170 g) zucchini noodles, made using a spiralizer or store-bought

1. Place the ground beef in a large bowl, and season with the salt.
2. Place the egg in a separate bowl and sprinkle with the gelatin. Allow to sit for 5 minutes.
3. Stir the gelatin mixture, then pour it over the ground beef. Add the Parmesan, garlic, and Italian seasoning. Season with salt and pepper.

4. Form the mixture into 1½-inch meatballs and place them on a plate; cover with plastic wrap and refrigerate for at least 1 hour or overnight.
5. Spray the meatballs with oil. Set the air fryer to 400°F (205°C) and arrange the meatballs in a single layer in the air fryer basket. Cook for 4 minutes. Flip the meatballs and spray them with more oil. Cook for 4 minutes more, until an instant-read thermometer reads 160°F (71°C). Transfer the meatballs to a plate and allow them to rest.
6. While the meatballs are resting, heat the marinara in a saucepan on the stove over medium heat.
7. Place the zucchini noodles in the air fryer, and cook at 400°F (205°C) for 3 to 5 minutes.
8. To serve, place the zucchini noodles in serving bowls. Top with meatballs and warm marinara.

Per Serving

calories: 312 | fat: 25g | protein: 20g | carbs: 2g | net carbs: 1g | fiber: 1g

Ribs with Chimichurri Sauce

Prep time: 15 minutes | Cook time: 13 minutes | Serves 4

1 pound (454 g) boneless short ribs

1½ teaspoons sea salt, divided

½ teaspoon freshly ground black pepper, divided

½ cup fresh parsley leaves

½ cup fresh cilantro leaves

1 teaspoon minced garlic

1 tablespoon freshly squeezed lemon juice

½ teaspoon ground cumin

¼ teaspoon red pepper flakes

2 tablespoons extra-virgin olive oil

Avocado oil spray

1. Pat the short ribs dry with paper towels. Sprinkle the ribs all over with 1 teaspoon salt and ¼ teaspoon black pepper. Let sit at room temperature for 45 minutes.
2. Meanwhile, place the parsley, cilantro, garlic, lemon juice, cumin, red pepper flakes, the remaining ½ teaspoon salt, and the remaining ¼ teaspoon black pepper in a blender or food processor. With the blender running, slowly drizzle in the olive oil. Blend for about 1 minute, until the mixture is smooth and well combined.

3. Set the air fryer to 400°F (205ºC). Spray both sides of the ribs with oil. Place in the basket and cook for 8 minutes. Flip and cook for another 5 minutes, until an instant-read thermometer reads 125°F (52ºC) for medium-rare (or to your desired doneness).
4. Allow the meat to rest for 5 to 10 minutes, then slice. Serve warm with the chimichurri sauce.

Per Serving

calories: 329 | fat: 24g | protein: 21g | carbs: 7g | net carbs: 6g | fiber: 1g

Spinach Cheese Steak

Prep time: 15 minutes | Cook time: 22 minutes | Serves 4

2 tablespoons balsamic vinegar

2 tablespoons red wine vinegar

1 tablespoon Dijon mustard

1 tablespoon Swerve or keto-friendly sweetener of choice

1 teaspoon minced garlic

Sea salt and freshly ground black pepper, to taste

¾ cup extra-virgin olive oil

1 pound (454 g) boneless sirloin steak

Avocado oil spray

1 small red onion, cut into ¼-inch-thick rounds

6 ounces (170 g) baby spinach

½ cup cherry tomatoes, halved

3 ounces (85 g) blue cheese, crumbled

1. In a blender, combine the balsamic vinegar, red wine vinegar, Dijon mustard, Swerve, and garlic. Season with salt and pepper and process until smooth. With the blender running, drizzle in the olive oil. Process until well combined. Transfer to a jar with a tight-fitting lid, and refrigerate until ready to serve (it will keep for up to 2 weeks).
2. Season the steak with salt and pepper and let sit at room temperature for at least 45 minutes, time permitting.
3. Set the air fryer to 400°F (205ºC). Spray the steak with oil and place it in the air fryer basket. Cook for 6 minutes. Flip the steak and spray it with more oil. Cook for 6 minutes more for medium-rare or until the steak is done to your liking.
4. Transfer the steak to a plate, tent with a piece of aluminum foil, and allow it to rest.

5. Spray the onion slices with oil and place them in the air fryer basket. Cook at 400°F (205ºC) for 5 minutes. Flip the onion slices and spray them with more oil. Cook for 5 minutes more.
6. Slice the steak diagonally into thin strips. Place the spinach, cherry tomatoes, onion slices, and steak in a large bowl. Toss with the desired amount of dressing. Sprinkle with crumbled blue cheese and serve.

Per Serving

calories: 670 | fat: 53g | protein: 41g | carbs: 9g | net carbs: 7g | fiber: 2g

Buttery Strip Steak

Prep time: 7 minutes | Cook time: 12 minutes | Serves 6

½ cup (1 stick) unsalted butter, at room temperature

1 cup finely grated Parmesan cheese

¼ cup finely ground blanched almond flour

1½ pounds (680g) New York strip steak

Sea salt, freshly ground black pepper, to taste

1. Place the butter, Parmesan cheese, and almond flour in a food processor. Process until smooth. Transfer to a sheet of parchment paper and form into a log. Wrap tightly in plastic wrap. Freeze for 45 minutes or refrigerate for at least 4 hours.
2. While the butter is chilling, season the steak liberally with salt and pepper. Let the steak rest at room temperature for about 45 minutes.
3. Place the grill pan or basket in your air fryer, set it to 400°F (205ºC), and let it preheat for 5 minutes.
4. Working in batches, if necessary, place the steak on the grill pan and cook for 4 minutes. Flip and cook for 3 minutes more, until the steak is brown on both sides.
5. Remove the steak from the air fryer and arrange an equal amount of the Parmesan butter on top of each steak. Return the steak to the air fryer and continue cooking for another 5 minutes, until an instant-read thermometer reads 120°F (49ºC) for medium-rare and the crust is golden brown (or to your desired doneness).
6. Transfer the cooked steak to a plate; let rest for 10 minutes before serving.

Per Serving

calories: 463 | fat: 37g | protein: 33g | carbs: 2g | net carbs: 1g | fiber: 1g

Steak with Butter

Prep time: 5 minutes | Cook time: 10 minutes | Serves 6

½ cup olive oil

2 tablespoons minced garlic

Sea salt, freshly ground black pepper, to taste

1½ pounds (680g) New York strip or top sirloin steak

Unsalted butter, for serving (optional)

1. In a bowl or blender, combine the olive oil, garlic, and salt and pepper to taste.
2. Place the steak in a shallow bowl or zip-top bag. Pour the marinade over the meat, seal, and marinate in the refrigerator for at least 1 hour and up to 24 hours.
3. Place a grill pan or basket in the air fryer, set it to 400°F (205ºC), and let preheat for 5 minutes.
4. Place the steak on the grill pan in a single layer, working in batches if necessary, and cook for 5 minutes. Flip the steak and cook for another 5 minutes, until an instant-read thermometer reads 120°F (49ºC) for medium-rare (or cook to your desired doneness).
5. Transfer the steak to a plate, and let rest for 10 minutes before serving. If desired, top the steaks with a pat of butter while they rest.

Per Serving

calories: 386 | fat: 32g | protein: 25g | carbs: 1g | net carbs: 1g | fiber: 0g

Steak with Bell Pepper

Prep time: 15 minutes | Cook time: 20 to 23 minutes | Serves 6

¼ cup avocado oil

¼ cup freshly squeezed lime juice

2 teaspoons minced garlic

1 tablespoon chili powder

½ teaspoon ground cumin

Sea salt, Freshly ground black pepper, to taste

1 pound (454 g) top sirloin steak or flank steak, thinly sliced against the grain

1 red bell pepper, cored, seeded, and cut into ½-inch slices

1 green bell pepper, cored, seeded, and cut into ½-inch slices

1 large onion, sliced

1. In a small bowl or blender, combine the avocado oil, lime juice, garlic, chili powder, cumin, and salt and pepper to taste.
2. Place the sliced steak in a zip-top bag or shallow dish. Place the bell peppers and onion in a separate zip-top bag or dish. Pour half the marinade over the steak and the other half over the vegetables. Seal both bags and let the steak and vegetables marinate in the refrigerator for at least 1 hour or up to 4 hours.
3. Line the air fryer basket with an air fryer liner or aluminum foil. Remove the vegetables from their bag or dish and shake off any excess marinade. Set the air fryer to 400°F (205ºC). Place the vegetables in the air fryer basket and cook for 13 minutes.
4. Remove the steak from its bag or dish and shake off any excess marinade. Place the steak on top of the vegetables in the air fryer, and cook for 7 to 10 minutes or until an instant-read thermometer reads 120°F (49ºC) for medium-rare (or cook to your desired doneness).
5. Serve with desired fixings, such as keto tortillas, lettuce, sour cream, avocado slices, shredded Cheddar cheese, and cilantro.

Per Serving

calories: 229 | fat: 14g | protein: 17g | carbs: 7g | net carbs: 5g | fiber: 2g

Cheesy Beef Burger with Mushroom

Prep time: 10 minutes | Cook time: 21 to 23 minutes | Serves 4

1 pound (454 g) ground beef, formed into 4 patties

Sea salt, freshly ground black pepper, to taste

1 cup thinly sliced onion

8 ounces (227 g) mushrooms, sliced

1 tablespoon avocado oil

2 ounces (57 g) Gruyère cheese, shredded (about ½ cup)

1. Season the patties on both sides with salt and pepper.
2. Set the air fryer to 375°F (190ºC). Place the patties in the basket and cook for 3 minutes. Flip and cook for another 2 minutes. Remove the burgers and set aside.

Place the onion and mushrooms in a medium bowl. Add the avocado oil and salt and pepper to taste; toss well.

3. Place the onion and mushrooms in the air fryer basket. Cook for 15 minutes, stirring occasionally.
4. Spoon the onions and mushrooms over the patties. Top with the cheese. Place the patties back in the air fryer basket and cook for another 1 to 3 minutes, until the cheese melts and an instant-read thermometer reads 160°F (71ºC). Remove and let rest. The temperature will rise to 165°F (74ºC), yielding a perfect medium-well burger.

Per Serving

calories: 470 | fat: 38g | protein: 25g | carbs: 5g | net carbs: 4g | fiber: 1g

Roast Beef

Prep time: 5 minutes | Cook time: 30 to 35 minutes | Serves 8

1 (2-pound / 907-g) top round beef roast, tied with kitchen string

Sea salt, Freshly ground black pepper, to taste

2 teaspoons minced garlic

2 tablespoons finely chopped fresh rosemary

¼ cup avocado oil

1. Season the roast generously with salt and pepper.
2. In a small bowl, whisk together the garlic, rosemary, and avocado oil. Rub this all over the roast. Cover loosely with aluminum foil or plastic wrap and refrigerate for at least 12 hours or up to 2 days.
3. Remove the roast from the refrigerator and allow to sit at room temperature for about 1 hour.
4. Set the air fryer to 325°F (163ºC). Place the roast in the air fryer basket and cook for 15 minutes. Flip the roast and cook for 15 to 20 minutes more, until the meat is browned and an instant-read thermometer reads 120°F (49ºC) at the thickest part (for medium-rare).
5. Transfer the meat to a cutting board, and let it rest for 15 minutes before thinly slicing and serving.

Per Serving

calories: 213 | fat: 10g | protein: 25g | carbs: 2g | net carbs: 1g | fiber: 1g

Beef Steak Shallots

Prep time: 5 minutes | Cook time: 18 to 20 minutes | Serves 6

1½ pounds (680g) beef tenderloin steaks

Sea salt, Freshly ground black pepper, to taste

4 medium shallots

1 teaspoon olive oil or avocado oil

1. Season both sides of the steaks with salt and pepper, and let them sit at room temperature for 45 minutes.
2. Set the air fryer to 400°F (205°C) and let it preheat for 5 minutes.
3. Working in batches if necessary, place the steaks in the air fryer basket in a single layer and cook for 5 minutes. Flip and cook for 5 minutes longer, until an instant-read thermometer inserted in the center of the steaks registers 120°F (49°C) for medium-rare (or as desired). Remove the steaks and tent with aluminum foil to rest.
4. Set the air fryer to 300°F (150°C). In a medium bowl, toss the shallots with the oil. Place the shallots in the basket and cook for 5 minutes, then give them a toss and cook for 3 to 5 minutes more, until crispy and golden brown.
5. Place the steaks on serving plates and arrange the shallots on top.

Per Serving

calories: 186 | fat: 5g | protein: 30g | carbs: 5g | net carbs: 5g | fiber: 0g

Steak with Horseradish Cream

Prep time: 5 minutes | Cook time: 10 minutes | Serves 8

2 pounds (907 g) rib eye steaks

Sea salt, Freshly ground black pepper, to taste

Unsalted butter, for serving

1 cup sour cream

$1/3$ cup heavy (whipping) cream

4 tablespoons prepared horseradish

1 teaspoon Dijon mustard

1 teaspoon apple cider vinegar

¼ teaspoon Swerve, to taste

1. Pat the steaks dry. Season with salt and pepper and let sit at room temperature for about 45 minutes.
2. Place the grill pan in the air fryer and set the air fryer to 400°F (205°C). Let preheat for 5 minutes.
3. Working in batches, place the steaks in a single layer on the grill pan and cook for 5 minutes. Flip the steaks and cook for 5 minutes more, until an instant-read thermometer reads 120°F (49°C) (or to your desired doneness).
4. Transfer the steaks to a plate and top each with a pat of butter. Tent with foil and let rest for 10 minutes.
5. Combine the sour cream, heavy cream, horseradish, Dijon mustard, vinegar, and Swerve in a bowl. Stir until smooth.
6. Serve the steaks with the horseradish cream.

Per Serving

calories: 322 | fat: 22g | protein: 23g | carbs: 6g | net carbs: 5g | fiber: 1g

Aromatic Ribeye Steak

Prep time: 20 minutes | Cook time: 15 minutes | Serves 3

1½ pounds (680g) ribeye, bone-in

1 tablespoon butter, room temperature

Salt, to taste

½ teaspoon crushed black pepper

½ teaspoon dried dill

½ teaspoon cayenne pepper

½ teaspoon garlic powder

½ teaspoon onion powder

1 teaspoon ground coriander

3 tablespoons mayonnaise

1 teaspoon garlic, minced

1. Start by preheating your Air Fryer to 400 degrees F (205°C).
2. Pat dry the ribeye and rub it with softened butter on all sides. Sprinkle with seasonings and transfer to the cooking basket.
3. Cook in the preheated Air Fryer for 15 minutes, flipping them halfway through the cooking time.

4. In the meantime, simply mix the mayonnaise with garlic and place in the refrigerator until ready to serve. Bon appétit!

Per Serving

calories: 437 | fat: 24g | protein: 51g | carbs: 2g | net carbs: 1g | fiber: 1g

Air Fried Top Chuck

Prep time: 15 minutes | Cook time: 50 minutes | Serves 3

1½ pounds (680g) top chuck

2 teaspoons olive oil

1 tablespoon Dijon mustard

Sea salt and ground black pepper, to taste

1 teaspoon dried marjoram

1 teaspoon dried thyme

½ teaspoon fennel seeds

1. Start by preheating your Air Fryer to 380 degrees F (193ºC)
2. Add all ingredients in a Ziploc bag; shake to mix well. Next, spritz the bottom of the Air Fryer basket with cooking spray.
3. Place the beef in the cooking basket and cook for 50 minutes, turning every 10 to 15 minutes.
4. Let it rest for 5 to 7 minutes before slicing and serving. Enjoy!

Per Serving

calories: 406 | fat: 24g | protein: 44g | carbs: 2 g | net carbs:1g | fiber: 1g

Beef Burger

Prep time: 20 minutes | Cook time: 12 minutes | Serves 4

1¼ pounds (567g) lean ground beef

1 tablespoon coconut aminos

1 teaspoon Dijon mustard

A few dashes of liquid smoke

1 teaspoon shallot powder

1 clove garlic, minced

½ teaspoon cumin powder

¼ cup scallions, minced

⅓ teaspoon sea salt flakes

⅓ teaspoon freshly cracked mixed peppercorns

1 teaspoon celery seeds

1 teaspoon parsley flakes

1. Mix all of the above ingredients in a bowl; knead until everything is well incorporated.
2. Shape the mixture into four patties. Next, make a shallow dip in the center of each patty to prevent them puffing up during air-frying.
3. Spritz the patties on all sides using a non-stick cooking spray. Cook approximately 12 minutes at 360 degrees F (182ºC).
4. Check for doneness – an instant read thermometer should read 160 degrees F (71ºC). Bon appétit!

Per Serving

calories: 425 | fat: 25g | protein: 38g | carbs: 10g | net carbs: 8g | fiber: 2g

Roast Beef

Prep time: 20 minutes | Cook time: 45 minutes | Serves 8

2 pounds (907 g) roast beef, at room temperature

2 tablespoons extra-virgin olive oil

1 teaspoon sea salt flakes

1 teaspoon black pepper, preferably freshly ground

1 teaspoon smoked paprika

A few dashes of liquid smoke

2 jalapeño peppers, thinly sliced

1. Start by preheating the Air Fryer to 330 degrees F (166ºC).
2. Then, pat the roast dry using kitchen towels. Rub with extra-virgin olive oil and all seasonings along with liquid smoke.
3. Roast for 30 minutes in the preheated Air Fryer; then, pause the machine and turn the roast over; roast for additional 15 minutes.

4. Check for doneness using a meat thermometer and serve sprinkled with sliced jalapeños. Bon appétit!

Per Serving

calories: 167 | fat: 5g | protein: 26g | carbs: 2g | net carbs: 1g | fiber: 1g

Roast Beef Steaks

Prep time: 20 minutes | Cook time: 20 minutes | Serves 4

2 tablespoons coconut aminos

3 heaping tablespoons fresh chives

2 tablespoons olive oil

3 tablespoons dry white wine

4 small-sized beef steaks

2 teaspoons smoked cayenne pepper

½ teaspoon dried basil

½ teaspoon dried rosemary

1 teaspoon freshly ground black pepper

1 teaspoon sea salt, or more to taste

1. Firstly, coat the steaks with the cayenne pepper, black pepper, salt, basil, and rosemary.
2. Drizzle the steaks with olive oil, white wine, and coconut aminos.
3. Finally, roast in an Air Fryer basket for 20 minutes at 335 degrees F (168ºC). Serve garnished with fresh chives. Bon appétit!

Per Serving

calories: 445 | fat: 23g | protein: 51g | carbs: 11g | net carbs: 10g | fiber: 1g

Air Fried Beef Steak

Prep time: 16 minutes | Cook time: 10 minutes | Serves 4

$1/3$ cup almond flour

2 eggs

2 teaspoons caraway seeds

4 beef steaks

2 teaspoons garlic powder

1 tablespoon melted butter

Fine sea salt and cayenne pepper, to taste

1. Generously coat steaks with garlic powder, caraway seeds, salt, and cayenne pepper.
2. In a mixing dish, thoroughly combine melted butter with seasoned crumbs. In another bowl, beat the eggs until they're well whisked.
3. First, coat steaks with the beaten egg; then, coat beef steaks with the buttered crumb mixture.
4. Place the steaks in the Air Fryer cooking basket; cook for 10 minutes at 355 degrees F (181ºC). Bon appétit!

Per Serving

calories: 474 | fat: 22g | protein: 55g | carbs: 9g | net carbs: 8g | fiber: 1g

Beef Parboiled Sausage

Prep time: 35 minutes | Cook time: 30 minutes | Serves 4

2 teaspoons olive oil

2 bell peppers, sliced

1 green bell pepper, sliced

1 serrano pepper, sliced

1 shallot, sliced

Sea salt and pepper, to taste

½ teaspoon dried thyme

1 teaspoon dried rosemary

½ teaspoon mustard seeds

1 teaspoon fennel seeds

2 pounds (907 g) thin beef parboiled sausage

1. Brush the sides and bottom of the cooking basket with 1 teaspoon of olive oil. Add the peppers and shallot to the cooking basket.
2. Toss them with the spices and cook at 390 degrees F (199ºC) for 15 minutes, shaking the basket occasionally. Reserve.
3. Turn the temperature to 380 degrees F (193ºC)
4. Then, add the remaining 1 teaspoon of oil. Once hot, add the sausage and cook in the preheated Air Frye for 15 minutes, flipping them halfway through the cooking time.
5. Serve with reserved pepper mixture. Bon appétit!

Per Serving

calories: 563 | fat: 41g | protein: 35g | carbs: 11g | net carbs: 10g | fiber: 1g

Red Wine Rib

Prep time: 20 minutes | Cook time: 10 minutes | Serves 4

1½ pounds (680g) short ribs

1 cup red wine

1 lemon, juiced

1 teaspoon fresh ginger, grated

1 teaspoon salt

1 teaspoon black pepper

1 teaspoon paprika

1 teaspoon chipotle chili powder

1 cup keto tomato paste

1 teaspoon garlic powder

1 teaspoon cumin

1. In a ceramic bowl, place the beef ribs, wine, lemon juice, ginger, salt, black pepper, paprika, and chipotle chili powder. Cover and let it marinate for 3 hours in the refrigerator.
2. Discard the marinade and add the short ribs to the Air Fryer basket. Cook in the preheated Air fry at 380 degrees F (193ºC) for 10 minutes, turning them over halfway through the cooking time.
3. In the meantime, heat the saucepan over medium heat; add the reserved marinade and stir in the tomato paste, garlic powder, and cumin. Cook until the sauce has thickened slightly.
4. Pour the sauce over the warm ribs and serve immediately. Bon appétit!

Per Serving

calories: 397 | fat: 15g | protein: 35g | carbs: 5g | net carbs: 4g | fiber: 1g

Chuck Kebab with Arugula

Prep time: 30 minutes | Cook time: 25 minutes | Serves 4

½ cup leeks, chopped

2 garlic cloves, smashed

2 pounds (907 g) ground chuck

Salt, to taste

¼ teaspoon ground black pepper, or more to taste

1 teaspoon cayenne pepper

½ teaspoon ground sumac

3 saffron threads

2 tablespoons loosely packed fresh continental parsley leaves

4 tablespoons tahini sauce

4 ounces (113 g) baby arugula

1 tomato, cut into slices

1. In a bowl, mix the chopped leeks, garlic, ground chuck, and spices; knead with your hands until everything is well incorporated.
2. Now, mound the beef mixture around a wooden skewer into a pointed-ended sausage.
3. Cook in the preheated Air Fryer at 360 degrees F (182ºC) for 25 minutes.
4. Serve your kebab with the tahini sauce baby arugula and tomato. Enjoy!

Per Serving

calories: 354 | fat: 15g | protein: 49g | carbs: 6g | net carbs: 4g | fiber: 2g

Cheesy Filet Mignon

Prep time: 20 minutes | Cook time: 13 minutes | Serves 4

1 pound (454 g) filet mignon

Sea salt and ground black pepper, to taste

½ teaspoon cayenne pepper

1 teaspoon dried basil

1 teaspoon dried rosemary

1 teaspoon dried thyme

1 tablespoon sesame oil

1 small-sized egg, well-whisked

½ cup Parmesan cheese, grated

1. Season the filet mignon with salt, black pepper, cayenne pepper, basil, rosemary, and thyme. Brush with sesame oil.
2. Put the egg in a shallow plate. Now, place the Parmesan cheese in another plate.
3. Coat the filet mignon with the egg; then, lay it into the Parmesan cheese. Set your Air Fryer to cook at 360 degrees F (182ºC).
4. Cook for 10 to 13 minutes or until golden. Serve with mixed salad leaves and enjoy!

Per Serving

calories: 315 | fat: 20g | protein: 30g | carbs: 4g | net carbs: 3g | fiber: 1g

Air Fried London Broil

Prep time: 30 minutes | Cook time: 8 to 10 minutes | Serves 8

2 pounds (907 g) London broil

3 large garlic cloves, minced

3 tablespoons balsamic vinegar

3 tablespoons whole-grain mustard

2 tablespoons olive oil

Sea salt and ground black pepper, to taste

½ teaspoon dried hot red pepper flakes

1. Score both sides of the cleaned London broil.
2. Thoroughly combine the remaining ingredients; massage this mixture into the meat to coat it on all sides. Let it marinate for at least 3 hours.
3. Set the Air Fryer to cook at 400 degrees F (205ºC); Then cook the London broil for 15 minutes. Flip it over and cook another 10 to 12 minutes. Bon appétit!

Per Serving

calories: 257 | fat: 9g | protein: 41g | carbs: 1g | net carbs: 0g | fiber: 1g

Creamy Beef Steak

Prep time: 20 minutes | Cook time: 15 minutes | Serves 4

1¼ pounds (567g) beef sirloin steak, cut into small-sized strips

¼ cup balsamic vinegar

1 tablespoon brown mustard

1 tablespoon butter

1 cup beef broth

1 cup leek, chopped

2 cloves garlic, crushed

1 teaspoon cayenne pepper

Sea salt flakes and crushed red pepper, to taste

1 cup sour cream

2½ tablespoons keto tomato paste

1. Place the beef along with the balsamic vinegar and the mustard in a mixing dish; cover and marinate in your refrigerator for about 1 hour.
2. Butter the inside of a baking dish and put the beef into the dish.
3. Add the broth, leeks and garlic. Cook at 380 degrees (193ºC) for 8 minutes. Pause the machine and add the cayenne pepper, salt, red pepper, sour cream and tomato paste; cook for additional 7 minutes.
4. Bon appétit!

Per Serving

calories: 418 | fat: 25g | protein: 33g | carbs: 9g | net carbs: 8g | fiber: 1g

Beef Chuck with Brussels Sprouts

Prep time: 30 minutes | Cook time: 25 minutes | Serves 4

1 pound (454 g) beef chuck shoulder steak

2 tablespoons olive oil

1 tablespoon red wine vinegar

1 teaspoon fine sea salt

½ teaspoon ground black pepper

1 teaspoon smoked paprika

1 teaspoon onion powder

½ teaspoon garlic powder

½ pound (227g) Brussels sprouts, cleaned and halved

½ teaspoon fennel seeds

1 teaspoon dried basil

1 teaspoon dried sage

1. Firstly, marinate the beef with olive oil, wine vinegar, salt, black pepper, paprika, onion powder, and garlic powder. Rub the marinade into the meat and let it stay at least for 3 hours.
2. Air fry at 390 degrees F (199ºC) for 10 minutes. Pause the machine and add the prepared Brussels sprouts; sprinkle them with fennel seeds, basil, and sage.
3. Turn the machine to 380 degrees F (193ºC); press the power button and cook for 5 more minutes. Pause the machine, stir and cook for further 10 minutes.
4. Next, remove the meat from the cooking basket and cook the vegetables a few minutes more if needed and according to your taste. Serve with your favorite mayo sauce.

Per Serving

calories: 272 | fat: 14g | protein: 26g | carbs: 6g | net carbs: 3g | fiber: 3g

Creamy Beef Flank Steak

Prep time: 13 minutes | Cook time: 7 minutes | Serves 2

1/3 cup sour cream

½ cup green onion, chopped

1 tablespoon mayonnaise

3 cloves garlic, smashed

1 pound (454 g) beef flank steak, trimmed and cubed

2 tablespoons fresh sage, minced

½ teaspoon salt

1/3 teaspoon black pepper, or to taste

1. Season your meat with salt and pepper; arrange beef cubes on the bottom of a baking dish that fits in your air fryer.
2. Stir in green onions and garlic; air-fry for about 7 minutes at 385 degrees F (196ºC).
3. Once your beef starts to tender, add the cream, mayonnaise, and sage; air-fry an additional 8 minutes. Bon appétit!

Per Serving

calories: 428 | fat: 20g | protein: 50g | carbs: 7g | net carbs: 6g | fiber: 1g

Air Fried Skirt Steak

Prep time: 20 minutes | Cook time: 12 minutes | Serves 5

2 pounds (907 g) skirt steak

2 tablespoons keto tomato paste

1 tablespoon olive oil

1 tablespoon coconut aminos

¼ cup rice vinegar

1 tablespoon fish sauce

Sea salt, to taste

½ teaspoon dried dill

½ teaspoon dried rosemary

¼ teaspoon black pepper, freshly cracked

1. Place all ingredients in a large ceramic dish; let it marinate for 3 hours in your refrigerator.
2. Coat the sides and bottom of the Air Fryer with cooking spray.
3. Add your steak to the cooking basket; reserve the marinade. Cook the skirt steak in the preheated Air Fryer at 400 degrees F (205ºC) for 12 minutes, turning over a couple of times, basting with the reserved marinade.
4. Bon appétit!

Per Serving

calories: 401 | fat: 21g | protein: 51g | carbs: 2g | net carbs: 1g | fiber: 1g

Beef Sausage with Tomato Bowl

Prep time: 35 minutes | Cook time: 20 minutes | Serves 4

4 bell peppers

2 tablespoons olive oil

2 medium-sized tomatoes, halved

4 spring onions

4 beef sausages

1 tablespoon mustard

1. Start by preheating your Air Fryer to 400 degrees F (205°C).
2. Add the bell peppers to the cooking basket. Drizzle 1 tablespoon of olive oil all over the bell peppers.
3. Cook for 5 minutes. Turn the temperature down to 350 degrees F (180°C). Add the tomatoes and spring onions to the cooking basket and cook an additional 10 minutes.
4. Reserve your vegetables.
5. Then, add the sausages to the cooking basket. Drizzle with the remaining tablespoon of olive oil.
6. Cook in the preheated Air Fryer at 380 degrees F (193°C) for 15 minutes, flipping them halfway through the cooking time.
7. Serve sausages with the air-fried vegetables and mustard; serve.

Per Serving

calories: 490 | fat: 42g | protein: 19g | carbs: 9g | net carbs: 7g | fiber: 2g

Loin Steak with Mayo

Prep time: 20 minutes | Cook time: 15 minutes | Serves 4

1 cup mayonnaise

1 tablespoon fresh rosemary, finely chopped

2 tablespoons Worcestershire sauce

Sea salt, to taste

½ teaspoon ground black pepper

1 teaspoon smoked paprika

1 teaspoon garlic, minced

1½ pounds (680g) short loin steak

1. Combine the mayonnaise, rosemary, Worcestershire sauce, salt, pepper, paprika, and garlic; mix to combine well.
2. Now, brush the mayonnaise mixture over both sides of the steak. Lower the steak onto the grill pan.
3. Grill in the preheated Air Fryer at 390 degrees F (199ºC) for 8 minutes. Turn the steaks over and grill an additional 7 minutes.
4. Check for doneness with a meat thermometer. Serve warm and enjoy!

Per Serving

calories: 620 | fat: 50g | protein: 40g | carbs: 3g | net carbs: 2g | fiber: 1g

Cheesy Sirloin Steak

Prep time: 20 minutes | Cook time: 14 minutes | Serves 4

1½ pounds (680g) sirloin steak

¼ cup red wine

¼ cup fresh lime juice

1 teaspoon garlic powder

1 teaspoon shallot powder

1 teaspoon celery seeds

1 teaspoon mustard seeds

Coarse sea salt and ground black pepper, to taste

1 teaspoon red pepper flakes

2 eggs, lightly whisked

1 cup Parmesan cheese

1 teaspoon paprika

1. Place the steak, red wine, lime juice, garlic powder, shallot powder, celery seeds, mustard seeds, salt, black pepper, and red pepper in a large ceramic bowl; let it marinate for 3 hours.
2. Tenderize the cube steak by pounding with a mallet; cut into 1-inch strips.
3. In a shallow bowl, whisk the eggs. In another bowl, mix the Parmesan cheese and paprika.
4. Dip the beef pieces into the whisked eggs and coat on all sides. Now, dredge the beef pieces in the Parmesan mixture.
5. Cook at 400 degrees F (205ºC) for 14 minutes, flipping halfway through the cooking time.
6. Meanwhile, make the sauce by heating the reserved marinade in a saucepan over medium heat; let it simmer until thoroughly warmed. Serve the steak fingers with the sauce on the side. Enjoy!

Per Serving

calories: 475 | fat: 26g | protein: 45g | carbs: 8g | net carbs: 7g | fiber: 1g

Lemony Beef Steak

Prep time: 25 minutes | Cook time: 18 minutes | Serves 2

1 pound (454 g) beef steaks

4 tablespoons white wine

2 teaspoons crushed coriander seeds

½ teaspoon fennel seeds

$1/3$ cup beef broth

2 tablespoons lemon zest, grated

2 tablespoons olive oil

½ lemon, cut into wedges

Salt flakes and freshly ground black pepper, to taste

1. Heat the oil in a saucepan over a moderate flame. Then, cook the garlic for 1 minute, or until just fragrant.
2. Remove the pan from the heat; add the beef broth, wine, lemon zest, coriander seeds, fennel, salt flakes, and freshly ground black. Pour the mixture into a baking dish.

3. Add beef steaks to the baking dish; toss to coat well. Now, tuck the lemon wedges among the beef steaks.
4. Bake for 18 minutes at 335 degrees F (168ºC). Serve warm.

Per Serving

calories: 447 | fat: 27g | protein: 48g | carbs: 3g | net carbs: 2g | fiber: 1g

Mushroom Sausage Biscuit

Prep time: 15 minutes | Cook time: 34 minutes | Serves 4

Filling:

1 pound (454 g) ground Italian sausage

1 cup sliced mushrooms

1 teaspoon fine sea salt

2 cups no-sugar-added marinara sauce

Biscuits:

3 large egg whites

¾ cup blanched almond flour

1 teaspoon baking powder

¼ teaspoon fine sea salt

2½ tablespoons very cold unsalted butter, cut into ¼-inch pieces

Fresh basil leaves, for garnish

1. Preheat the air fryer to 400°F (205ºC).
2. Place the sausage in a 7-inch pie pan (or a pan that fits into your air fryer). Use your hands to break up the sausage and spread it evenly on the bottom of the pan. Place the pan in the air fryer and cook for 5 minutes.
3. Remove the pan from the air fryer and use a fork or metal spatula to crumble the sausage more. Season the mushrooms with the salt and add them to the pie pan. Stir to combine the mushrooms and sausage, then return the pan to the air fryer and cook for 4 minutes, or until the mushrooms are soft and the sausage is cooked through.
4. Remove the pan from the air fryer. Add the marinara sauce and stir well. Set aside.
5. Make the biscuits: Place the egg whites in a large mixing bowl or the bowl of a stand mixer. Using a hand mixer or stand mixer, whip the egg whites until stiff peaks form.
6. In a medium-sized bowl, whisk together the almond flour, baking powder, and salt, then cut in the butter. Gently fold the flour mixture into the egg whites with a rubber spatula.

7. Using a large spoon or ice cream scoop, spoon one-quarter of the dough on top of the sausage mixture, making sure the butter stays in separate clumps. Repeat with the remaining dough, spacing the biscuits about 1-inch apart.
8. Place the pan in the air fryer and cook for 5 minutes, then lower the heat to 325°F (163°C) and cook for another 15 to 20 minutes, until the biscuits are golden brown. Serve garnished with fresh basil leaves.
9. Store leftovers in an airtight container in the refrigerator for up to 3 days. Reheat in a preheated 350°F (180°C) air fryer for 5 minutes, or until warmed through.

Per Serving

calories: 588 | fat: 48g | protein: 28g | carbs: 9g | net carbs: 6g | fiber: 3g

Cheesy Sausage Balls

Prep time: 10 minutes | Cook time: 10 minutes | Serves 12

1¾ cups finely ground blanched almond flour

1 tablespoon baking powder

½ teaspoon sea salt

¼ teaspoon freshly ground black pepper

¼ teaspoon cayenne pepper

1 pound (454 g) fresh pork sausage, casings removed, crumbled

8 ounces (227 g) Cheddar cheese, shredded

8 ounces (227 g) cream cheese, at room temperature, cut into chunks

1. In a large mixing bowl, combine the almond flour, baking powder, salt, black pepper, and cayenne pepper.
2. Add the sausage, Cheddar cheese, and cream cheese. Stir to combine, and then, using clean hands, mix until all of the ingredients are well incorporated.
3. Form the mixture into 1½-inch balls.
4. Set the air fryer to 350°F (180°C). Arrange the sausage balls in a single layer in the air fryer basket, working in batches if necessary. Cook for 5 minutes. Flip the sausage balls and cook for 5 minutes more.

Per Serving

calories: 386 | fat: 27g | protein: 16g | carbs: 5g | net carbs: 3g | fiber: 2g

Italian Sausage Link

Prep time: 10 minutes | Cook time: 24minutes | Serves 4

1 bell pepper (any color), sliced

1 medium onion, sliced

1 tablespoon avocado oil

1 teaspoon Italian seasoning

Sea salt, Freshly ground black pepper, to taste

1 pound (454 g) Italian sausage links

1. Place the bell pepper and onion in a medium bowl, and toss with the avocado oil, Italian seasoning, and salt and pepper to taste.
2. Set the air fryer to 400°F (205ºC). Put the vegetables in the air fryer basket and cook for 12 minutes.
3. Push the vegetables to the side of the basket and arrange the sausage links in the bottom of the basket in a single layer. Spoon the vegetables over the sausages. Cook for 12 minutes, tossing halfway through, until an instant-read thermometer inserted into the sausage reads 160°F (71ºC).

Per Serving

calories: 339 | fat: 27g | protein: 17g | carbs: 5g | net carbs: 4g | fiber: 1g

Cheese Pork Chop

Prep time: 15 minutes | Cook time: 9 to 14 minutes | Serves 4

2 large eggs

½ cup finely grated Parmesan cheese

½ cup finely ground blanched almond flour or finely crushed pork rinds

1 teaspoon paprika

½ teaspoon dried oregano

½ teaspoon garlic powder

Salt, Freshly ground black pepper, to taste

1¼ pounds (567g) (1-inch-thick) boneless pork chops

Avocado oil spray

1. Beat the eggs in a shallow bowl. In a separate bowl, combine the Parmesan cheese, almond flour, paprika, oregano, garlic powder, and salt and pepper to taste.
2. Dip the pork chops into the eggs, then coat them with the Parmesan mixture, gently pressing the coating onto the meat. Spray the breaded pork chops with oil.
3. Set the air fryer to 400°F. Place the pork chops in the air fryer basket in a single layer, working in batches if necessary. Cook for 6 minutes. Flip the chops and spray them with more oil. Cook for another 3 to 8 minutes, until an instant-read thermometer reads 145°F (63ºC).
4. Allow the pork chops to rest for at least 5 minutes, then serve.

Per Serving

calories: 351 | fat: 20g | protein: 38g | carbs: 4g | net carbs: 2g | fiber: 2g

Bacon-Wrapped Cheese Pork

Prep time: 10 minutes | Cook time: 20 minutes | Serves 4

4 (1-inch-thick) boneless pork chops

2 (5.2-ounce / 147 g) packages Boursin cheese (or Kite Hill brand chive cream cheese style spread, softened, for dairy-free)

8 slices thin-cut bacon

1. Spray the air fryer basket with avocado oil. Preheat the air fryer to 400°F (205ºC).
2. Place one of the chops on a cutting board. With a sharp knife held parallel to the cutting board, make a 1-inch-wide incision on the top edge of the chop. Carefully cut into the chop to form a large pocket, leaving a ½-inch border along the sides and bottom. Repeat with the other 3 chops.
3. Snip the corner of a large resealable plastic bag to form a ¾-inch hole. Place the Boursin cheese in the bag and pipe the cheese into the pockets in the chops, dividing the cheese evenly among them.
4. Wrap 2 slices of bacon around each chop and secure the ends with toothpicks. Place the bacon-wrapped chops in the air fryer basket and cook for 10 minutes, then flip the chops and cook for another 8 to 10 minutes, until the bacon is crisp, the chops are cooked through, and the internal temperature reaches 145°F (63ºC).
5. Store leftovers in an airtight container in the refrigerator for up to 3 days. Reheat in a preheated 400°F (205ºC) air fryer for 5 minutes, or until warmed through.

Per Serving

calories: 578 | fat: 45g | protein: 37g | carbs: 16g | net carbs: 15g | fiber: 1g

Pork with Lime Sauce

Prep time: 10 minutes | Cook time: 15 minutes | Serves 4

Marinade:

½ cup lime juice

Grated zest of 1 lime

2 teaspoons stevia glycerite, or ¼ teaspoon liquid stevia

3 cloves garlic, minced

1½ teaspoons fine sea salt

1 teaspoon chili powder, or more for more heat

1 teaspoon smoked paprika

1 pound (454 g) pork tenderloin

Avocado Lime Sauce:

1 medium-sized ripe avocado, roughly chopped

½ cup full-fat sour cream (or coconut cream for dairy-free)

Grated zest of 1 lime

Juice of 1 lime

2 cloves garlic, roughly chopped

½ teaspoon fine sea salt

¼ teaspoon ground black pepper

Chopped fresh cilantro leaves, for garnish

Lime slices, for serving

Pico de gallo, for serving

1. In a medium-sized casserole dish, stir together all the marinade ingredients until well combined. Add the tenderloin and coat it well in the marinade. Cover and place in the fridge to marinate for 2 hours or overnight.
2. Spray the air fryer basket with avocado oil. Preheat the air fryer to 400°F (205ºC).
3. Remove the pork from the marinade and place it in the air fryer basket. Cook for 13 to 15 minutes, until the internal temperature of the pork is 145°F (63ºC), flipping after 7 minutes. Remove the pork from the air fryer and place it on a cutting board. Allow it to rest for 8 to 10 minutes, then cut it into ½-inch-thick slices.
4. While the pork cooks, make the avocado lime sauce: Place all the sauce ingredients in a food processor and purée until smooth. Taste and adjust the seasoning to your liking.
5. Place the pork slices on a serving platter and spoon the avocado lime sauce on top. Garnish with cilantro leaves and serve with lime slices and pico de gallo.

6. Store leftovers in an airtight container in the fridge for up to 4 days. Reheat in a preheated 400°F (205ºC) air fryer for 5 minutes, or until heated through.

Per Serving

calories: 326 | fat: 19g | protein: 26g | carbs: 15g | net carbs: 9g | fiber: 6g

Air Fried Pork Belly

Prep time: 10 minutes | Cook time: 17 minutes | Serves 4

1 pound (454 g) unsalted pork belly

2 teaspoons Chinese five-spice powder

Sauce:

1 tablespoon coconut oil

1 (1-inch) piece fresh ginger, peeled and grated

2 cloves garlic, minced

½ cup beef or chicken broth

¼ to ½ cup Swerve confectioners'-style sweetener or equivalent amount of liquid or powdered sweetener

3 tablespoons wheat-free tamari, or ½ cup coconut aminos

1 green onion, sliced, plus more for garnish

1. Spray the air fryer basket with avocado oil. Preheat the air fryer to 400°F (205ºC).
2. Cut the pork belly into ½-inch-thick slices and season well on all sides with the five-spice powder. Place the slices in a single layer in the air fryer basket (if you're using a smaller air fryer, work in batches if necessary) and cook for 8 minutes, or until cooked to your liking, flipping halfway through.
3. While the pork belly cooks, make the sauce: Heat the coconut oil in a small saucepan over medium heat. Add the ginger and garlic and sauté for 1 minute, or until fragrant. Add the broth, sweetener, and tamari and simmer for 10 to 15 minutes, until thickened. Add the green onion and cook for another minute, until the green onion is softened. Taste and adjust the seasoning to your liking.
4. Transfer the pork belly to a large bowl. Pour the sauce over the pork belly and coat well. Place the pork belly slices on a serving platter and garnish with sliced green onions.
5. Best served fresh. Store leftovers in an airtight container in the fridge for up to 4 days. Reheat in a preheated 400°F (205ºC) air fryer for 3 minutes, or until heated through.

Per Serving

calories: 365 | fat: 32g | protein: 19g | carbs: 2g | net carbs: 1g | fiber: 1g

Roast Pork Belly

Prep time: 20 minutes | Cook time: 30 minutes | Serves 6

1½ pounds (680g) pork belly

2 bell peppers, sliced

2 cloves garlic, finely minced

4 green onions, quartered, white and green parts

¼ cup cooking wine

Kosher salt and ground black pepper, to taste

1 teaspoon cayenne pepper

1 tablespoon coriander

1 teaspoon celery seeds

1. Blanch the pork belly in boiling water for approximately 15 minutes. Then, cut it into chunks.
2. Arrange the pork chunks, bell peppers, garlic, and green onions in the Air Fryer basket. Drizzle everything with cooking wine of your choice.
3. Sprinkle with salt, black pepper, cayenne pepper, fresh coriander, and celery seeds. Toss to coat well.
4. Roast in the preheated Air Fryer at 330 degrees (166ºC) F for 30 minutes.
5. Serve on individual serving plates. Bon appétit!

Per Serving

calories: 589 | fat: 60g | protein: 12g | carbs: 3g | net carbs: 2g | fiber: 1g

Air Fried Pork Meatballs

Prep time: 20 minutes | Cook time: 15 minutes | Serves 4

1 pound (454 g) ground pork

1 cup scallions, finely chopped

2 cloves garlic, finely minced

1½ tablespoons Worcester sauce

1 tablespoon coconut aminos

1 teaspoon turmeric powder

½ teaspoon freshly grated ginger root

1 small sliced red chili, for garnish

1. Mix all of the above ingredients, apart from the red chili. Knead with your hands to ensure an even mixture.
2. Roll into equal balls and transfer them to the Air Fryer cooking basket.
3. Set the timer for 15 minutes and push the power button. Air-fry at 350 degrees F (180ºC). Sprinkle with sliced red chili; serve immediately with your favorite sauce for dipping. Enjoy!

Per Serving

calories: 506 | fat: 42g | protein: 24g | carbs: 7g | net carbs: 5g | fiber: 2g

Onion Pork Kebabs

Prep time: 22 minutes | Cook time: 18 minutes | Serves 3

2 tablespoons tomato purée

½ fresh serrano, minced

1/3 teaspoon paprika

1 pound (454 g) pork, ground

½ cup green onions, finely chopped

3 cloves garlic, peeled and finely minced

1 teaspoon ground black pepper, or more to taste

1 teaspoon salt, or more to taste

1. Thoroughly combine all ingredients in a mixing dish. Then, form your mixture into sausage shapes.
2. Cook for 18 minutes at 355 degrees F (181ºC). Mound salad on a serving platter, top with air-fried kebabs and serve warm. Bon appétit!

Per Serving

calories: 413 | fat: 32g | protein: 26g | carbs: 3g | net carbs: 2g | fiber: 1g

Pork Kebab with Yogurt Sauce

Prep time: 25 minutes | Cook time: 12 minutes | Serves 4

2 teaspoons olive oil

½ pound (227g) ground pork

½ pound (227g) ground beef

1 egg, whisked

Sea salt and ground black pepper, to taste

1 teaspoon paprika

2 garlic cloves, minced

1 teaspoon dried marjoram

1 teaspoon mustard seeds

½ teaspoon celery seeds

Yogurt Sauce:

2 tablespoons olive oil

2 tablespoons fresh lemon juice

Sea salt, to taste

¼ teaspoon red pepper flakes, crushed

½ cup full-fat yogurt

1 teaspoon dried dill weed

1. Spritz the sides and bottom of the cooking basket with 2 teaspoons of olive oil.
2. In a mixing dish, thoroughly combine the ground pork, beef, egg, salt, black pepper, paprika, garlic, marjoram, mustard seeds, and celery seeds.
3. Form the mixture into kebabs and transfer them to the greased cooking basket. Cook at 365 degrees F (185ºC) for 11 to 12 minutes, turning them over once or twice.
4. In the meantime, mix all the sauce ingredients and place in the refrigerator until ready to serve. Serve the pork kebabs with the yogurt sauce on the side. Enjoy!

Per Serving

calories: 407 | fat: 29g | protein: 33g | carbs: 4g | net carbs: 3g | fiber: 1g

Cheesy Pork Beef Casserole

Prep time: 20 minutes | Cook time: 10 minutes | Serves 4

1 pound (454 g) lean ground pork

½ pound (227g) ground beef

¼ cup tomato purée

Sea salt and ground black pepper, to taste

1 teaspoon smoked paprika

½ teaspoon dried oregano

1 teaspoon dried basil

1 teaspoon dried rosemary

2 eggs

1 cup Cottage cheese, crumbled, at room temperature

½ cup Cotija cheese, shredded

1. Lightly grease a casserole dish with a nonstick cooking oil. Add the ground meat to the bottom of your casserole dish.
2. Add the tomato purée. Sprinkle with salt, black pepper, paprika, oregano, basil, and rosemary.
3. In a mixing bowl, whisk the egg with cheese. Place on top of the ground meat mixture. Place a piece of foil on top.
4. Bake in the preheated Air Fryer at 350 degrees F (180ºC) for 10 minutes; remove the foil and cook an additional 6 minutes. Bon appétit!

Per Serving

calories: 449 | fat: 23g | protein: 54g | carbs: 5g | net carbs: 4g | fiber: 1g

Savory Porterhouse Steak

Prep time: 20 minutes | Cook time: 14 minutes | Serves 2

1 pound (454 g) porterhouse steak, cut meat from bones in 2 pieces

½ teaspoon ground black pepper

1 teaspoon cayenne pepper

½ teaspoon salt

1 teaspoon garlic powder

½ teaspoon dried thyme

½ teaspoon dried marjoram

1 teaspoon Dijon mustard

1 tablespoon butter, melted

1. Sprinkle the porterhouse steak with all the seasonings.
2. Spread the mustard and butter evenly over the meat.
3. Cook in the preheated Air Fryer at 390 degrees F (199ºC) for 12 to 14 minutes.
4. Taste for doneness with a meat thermometer and serve immediately.

Per Serving

calories: 402 | fat: 14g | protein: 67g | carbs: 2g | net carbs: 1g | fiber: 1g

Cheese Wine Pork Cutlets

Prep time: 20 minutes | Cook time: 15 minutes | Serves 2

1 cup water

1 cup red wine

1 tablespoon sea salt

2 pork cutlets

¼ cup almond meal

¼ cup flaxseed meal

½ teaspoon baking powder

1 teaspoon shallot powder

½ teaspoon porcini powder

Sea salt and ground black pepper, to taste

1 egg

¼ cup yogurt

1 teaspoon brown mustard

$1/3$ cup Parmesan cheese, grated

1. In a large ceramic dish, combine the water, wine and salt. Add the pork cutlets and put for 1 hour in the refrigerator.

2. In a shallow bowl, mix the almond meal, flaxseed meal, baking powder, shallot powder, porcini powder, salt, and ground pepper. In another bowl, whisk the eggs with yogurt and mustard.
3. In a third bowl, place the grated Parmesan cheese.
4. Dip the pork cutlets in the seasoned flour mixture and toss evenly; then, in the egg mixture. Finally, roll them over the grated Parmesan cheese.
5. Spritz the bottom of the cooking basket with cooking oil. Add the breaded pork cutlets and cook at 395 degrees F (202ºC) and for 10 minutes.
6. Flip and cook for 5 minutes more on the other side. Serve warm.

Per Serving

calories: 450 | fat: 26g | protein: 41g | carbs: 9g | net carbs: 7g | fiber: 2g

Cheesy Pork Tenderloin

Prep time: 25 minutes | Cook time: 22 minutes | Serves 4

2 tablespoons olive oil
2 pounds (907 g) pork tenderloin, cut into serving-size pieces
1 teaspoon coarse sea salt
½ teaspoon freshly ground pepper
¼ teaspoon chili powder
1 teaspoon dried marjoram
1 tablespoon mustard
1 cup Ricotta cheese
1½ cups chicken broth

1. Start by preheating your Air Fryer to 350 degrees F (180ºC).
2. Heat the olive oil in a pan over medium-high heat. Once hot, cook the pork for 6 to 7 minutes, flipping it to ensure even cooking.
3. Arrange the pork in a lightly greased casserole dish. Season with salt, black pepper, chili powder, and marjoram.
4. In a mixing dish, thoroughly combine the mustard, cheese, and chicken broth. Pour the mixture over the pork chops in the casserole dish.
5. Bake for another 15 minutes or until bubbly and heated through. Bon appétit!

Per Serving

calories: 433 | fat: 20g | protein: 56g | carbs: 3g | net carbs: 2g | fiber: 1g

Cheese Pork Meatballs

Prep time: 15 minutes | Cook time: 7 minutes | Serves 3

1 pound (454 g) ground pork

1 tablespoon coconut aminos

1 teaspoon garlic, minced

2 tablespoons spring onions, finely chopped

½ cup pork rinds

½ cup Parmesan cheese, preferably freshly grated

1. Combine the ground pork, coconut aminos, garlic, and spring onions in a mixing dish. Mix until everything is well incorporated.
2. Form the mixture into small meatballs.
3. In a shallow bowl, mix the pork rinds and grated Parmesan cheese. Roll the meatballs over the Parmesan mixture.
4. Cook at 380 degrees F (193ºC) for 3 minutes; shake the basket and cook an additional 4 minutes or until meatballs are browned on all sides. Bon appétit!

Per Serving

calories: 539 | fat: 43g | protein: 32g | carbs: 3g | net carbs: 2g | fiber: 1g

Air Fried Pork Chop

Prep time: 22 minutes | Cook time: 18 minutes | Serves 6

2 tablespoons vermouth

6 center-cut loin pork chops

½ tablespoon fresh basil, minced

$1/3$ teaspoon freshly ground black pepper, or more to taste

2 tablespoons whole grain mustard

1 teaspoon fine kosher salt

1. Toss pork chops with other ingredients until they are well coated on both sides.

2. Air-fry your chops for 18 minutes at 405 degrees F (207ºC), turning once or twice.
3. Mound your favorite salad on a serving plate; top with pork chops and enjoy.

Per Serving

calories: 393 | fat: 15g | protein: 56g | carbs: 3g | net carbs: 2g | fiber: 1g

Roast Pork Tenderloin

Prep time: 20 minutes | Cook time: 17 minutes | Serves 4

1 pound (454 g) pork tenderloin
4-5 garlic cloves, peeled and halved
1 teaspoon kosher salt
$1/3$ teaspoon ground black pepper
1 teaspoon dried basil
½ teaspoon dried oregano
½ teaspoon dried rosemary
½ teaspoon dried marjoram
2 tablespoons cooking wine

1. Rub the pork with garlic halves; add the seasoning and drizzle with the cooking wine. Then, cut slits completely through pork tenderloin. Tuck the remaining garlic into the slits.
2. Wrap the pork tenderloin with foil; let it marinate overnight.
3. Roast at 360 degrees F (182ºC) for 15 to 17 minutes. Serve warm.

Per Serving

calories: 168 | fat: 4g | protein: 30g | carbs: 2g | net carbs: 1g | fiber: 1g

Aromatic Pork Loin Roast

Prep time: 55 minutes | Cook time: 55 minutes | Serves 6

1½ pounds (680g) boneless pork loin roast, washed
1 teaspoon mustard seeds
1 teaspoon garlic powder

1 teaspoon porcini powder

1 teaspoon shallot powder

¾ teaspoon sea salt flakes

1 teaspoon red pepper flakes, crushed

2 dried sprigs thyme, crushed

2 tablespoons lime juice

1. Firstly, score the meat using a small knife; make sure to not cut too deep.
2. In a small-sized mixing dish, combine all seasonings in the order listed above; mix to combine well.
3. Massage the spice mix into the pork meat to evenly distribute. Drizzle with lemon juice.
4. Then, set your Air Fryer to cook at 360 degrees F (182ºC). Place the pork in the Air Fryer basket; roast for 25 to 30 minutes. Pause the machine, check for doneness and cook for 25 minutes more.

Per Serving

calories: 278 | fat: 16g | protein: 31g | carbs: 2g | net carbs: 1g | fiber: 1g

Savory Pork Loin

Prep time: 50 minutes | Cook time: 16 minutes | Serves 3

1 teaspoon Celtic sea salt

½ teaspoon black pepper, freshly cracked

¼ cup red wine

2 tablespoons mustard

2 garlic cloves, minced

1 pound (454 g) pork top loin

1 tablespoon Italian herb seasoning blend

1. In a ceramic bowl, mix the salt, black pepper, red wine, mustard, and garlic. Add the pork top loin and let it marinate at least 30 minutes.
2. Spritz the sides and bottom of the cooking basket with a nonstick cooking spray.
3. Place the pork top loin in the basket; sprinkle with the Italian herb seasoning blend.
4. Cook the pork tenderloin at 370 degrees F (188ºC) for 10 minutes. Flip halfway through, spraying with cooking oil and cook for 5 to 6 minutes more. Serve immediately.

Per Serving

calories: 300 | fat: 9g | protein: 34g | carbs: 2g | net carbs: 1g | fiber: 1g

Greens with Shallot and Bacon

Prep time: 10 minutes | Cook time: 7 minutes | Serves 2

7 ounces (198 g) mixed greens

8 thick slices pork bacon

2 shallots, peeled and diced

Nonstick cooking spray

1. Begin by preheating the air fryer to 345 degrees F (174ºC).
2. Now, add the shallot and bacon to the Air Fryer cooking basket; set the timer for 2 minutes. Spritz with a nonstick cooking spray.
3. After that, pause the Air Fryer; throw in the mixed greens; give it a good stir and cook an additional 5 minutes. Serve warm.

Per Serving

calories: 259 | fat: 16g | protein: 19g | carbs: 10g | net carbs: 5g | fiber: 5g

Cheesy Pork Sausage Meatball

Prep time: 20 minutes | Cook time: 10 minutes | Serves 4

1 pound (454 g) pork sausage meat

1 shallot, finely chopped

2 garlic cloves, finely minced

½ teaspoon fine sea salt

¼ teaspoon ground black pepper, or more to taste

¾ teaspoon paprika

½ cup Parmesan cheese, preferably freshly grated

½ jar no-sugar-added marinara sauce

1. Mix all of the above ingredients, except the marinara sauce, in a large-sized dish, until everything is well incorporated.

2. Shape into meatballs. Air-fry them at 360 degrees F (182ºC) for 10 minutes; pause the Air Fryer, shake them up and cook for additional 6 minutes or until the balls are no longer pink in the middle.
3. Meanwhile, heat the marinara sauce over a medium flame. Serve the pork sausage meatballs with marinara sauce. Bon appétit!

Per Serving

calories: 409 | fat: 33g | protein: 17g | carbs: 7g | net carbs: 6g | fiber: 1g

Pork Cheese Casserole

Prep time: 50 minutes | Cook time: 30 minutes | Serves 4

2 chili peppers

1 red bell pepper

2 tablespoons olive oil

1 large-sized shallot, chopped

1 pound (454 g) ground pork

2 garlic cloves, minced

2 ripe tomatoes, puréed

1 teaspoon dried marjoram

½ teaspoon mustard seeds

½ teaspoon celery seeds

1 teaspoon Mexican oregano

1 tablespoon fish sauce

2 tablespoons fresh coriander, chopped

Salt and ground black pepper, to taste

2 cups water

1 tablespoon chicken bouillon granules

2 tablespoons sherry wine

1 cup Mexican cheese blend

1. Roast the peppers in the preheated Air Fryer at 395 degrees F (202ºC) for 10 minutes, flipping them halfway through cook time.
2. Let them steam for 10 minutes; then, peel the skin and discard the stems and seeds. Slice the peppers into halves.

3. Heat the olive oil in a baking pan at 380 degrees F (193ºC) for 2 minutes; add the shallots and cook for 4 minutes. Add the ground pork and garlic; cook for a further 4 to 5 minutes.
4. After that, stir in the tomatoes, marjoram, mustard seeds, celery seeds, oregano, fish sauce, coriander, salt, and pepper. Add a layer of sliced peppers to the baking pan.
5. Mix the water with the chicken bouillon granules and sherry wine. Add the mixture to the baking pan.
6. Cook in the preheated Air Fryer at 395 degrees F (202ºC) for 10 minutes. Top with cheese and bake an additional 5 minutes until the cheese has melted. Serve immediately.

Per Serving

calories: 505 | fat: 39g | protein: 28g | carbs: 10g | net carbs: 8g | fiber: 2g

Baked Sauerkraut with Sausage

Prep time: 35 minutes | Cook time: 16 minutes | Serves 4

4 pork sausages, smoked

2 tablespoons olive oil

2 garlic cloves, minced

1 pound (454 g) sauerkraut

1 teaspoon cayenne pepper

½ teaspoon black peppercorns

2 bay leaves

1. Start by preheating your Air Fryer to 360 degrees F (182ºC).
2. Prick holes into the sausages using a fork and transfer them to the cooking basket. Cook approximately 14 minutes, shaking the basket a couple of times. Set aside.
3. Now, heat the olive oil in a baking pan at 380 degrees F (193ºC). Add the garlic and cook for 1 minute. Immediately stir in the sauerkraut, cayenne pepper, peppercorns, and bay leaves.
4. Let it cook for 15 minutes, stirring every 5 minutes. Serve in individual bowls with warm sausages on the side!

Per Serving

calories: 453 | fat: 42g | protein: 17g | carbs: 6g | net carbs: 3g | fiber: 3g

Greek Pork with Tzatziki Sauce

Prep time: 55 minutes | Cook time: 50 minutes | Serves 4

Greek Pork:

2 pounds (907 g) pork sirloin roast

Salt and black pepper, to taste

1 teaspoon smoked paprika

½ teaspoon mustard seeds

½ teaspoon celery seeds

1 teaspoon fennel seeds

1 teaspoon Ancho chili powder

1 teaspoon turmeric powder

½ teaspoon ground ginger

2 tablespoons olive oil

2 cloves garlic, finely chopped

Tzatziki:

½ cucumber, finely chopped and squeezed

1 cup full-fat Greek yogurt

1 garlic clove, minced

1 tablespoon extra virgin olive oil

1 teaspoon balsamic vinegar

1 teaspoon minced fresh dill

A pinch of salt

1. Toss all ingredients for Greek pork in a large mixing bowl. Toss until the meat is well coated.
2. Cook in the preheated Air Fryer at 360 degrees F (182ºC) for 30 minutes; turn over and cook another 20 minutes.
3. Meanwhile, prepare the tzatziki by mixing all the tzatziki ingredients. Place in your refrigerator until ready to use.
4. Serve the pork sirloin roast with the chilled tzatziki on the side. Enjoy!

Per Serving

calories: 560 | fat: 30g | protein: 64g | carbs: 5g | net carbs: 3g | fiber: 2g

Tangy Lamb Chop

Prep time: 5 minutes | Cook time: 5 minutes | Serves 2

Marinade:

2 teaspoons grated lime zest
½ cup lime juice
¼ cup avocado oil
¼ cup chopped fresh mint leaves
4 cloves garlic, roughly chopped
2 teaspoons fine sea salt
½ teaspoon ground black pepper
4 (1-inch-thick) lamb chops
Sprigs of fresh mint, for garnish (optional)
Lime slices, for serving (optional)

1. Make the marinade: Place all the ingredients for the marinade in a food processor or blender and purée until mostly smooth with a few small chunks. Transfer half of the marinade to a shallow dish and set the other half aside for serving. Add the lamb to the shallow dish, cover, and place in the refrigerator to marinate for at least 2 hours or overnight.
2. Spray the air fryer basket with avocado oil. Preheat the air fryer to 390°F (199ºC).
3. Remove the chops from the marinade and place them in the air fryer basket. Cook for 5 minutes, or until the internal temperature reaches 145°F for medium doneness.
4. Allow the chops to rest for 10 minutes before serving with the rest of the marinade as a sauce. Garnish with fresh mint leaves and serve with lime slices, if desired. Best served fresh.

Per Serving

calories: 692 | fat: 53g | protein: 48g | carbs: 2g | net carbs: 1g | fiber: 1g

Fish and Seafood

Air Fried Fish Fillet

Prep time: 5 minutes | Cook time: 7 minutes | Serves 4

1 pound (454 g) snapper, grouper, or salmon fillets

Sea salt, freshly ground black pepper, to taste

1 tablespoon avocado oil

¼ cup sour cream

¼ cup sugar-free mayonnaise (homemade, here, or store-bought)

2 tablespoons fresh dill, chopped, plus more for garnish

1 tablespoon freshly squeezed lemon juice

½ teaspoon grated lemon zest

1. Pat the fish dry with paper towels and season well with salt and pepper. Brush with the avocado oil.
2. Set the air fryer to 400°F (205ºC). Place the fillets in the air fryer basket and cook for 1 minute.
3. Lower the air fryer temperature to 325°F and continue cooking for 5 minutes. Flip the fish and cook for 1 minute more or until an instant-read thermometer reads 145°F (63ºC). (If using salmon, cook it to 125°F (52ºC) for medium-rare.)
4. While the fish is cooking, make the sauce by combining the sour cream, mayonnaise, dill, lemon juice, and lemon zest in a medium bowl. Season with salt and pepper and stir until combined. Refrigerate until ready to serve.
5. Serve the fish with the sauce, garnished with the remaining dill.

Per Serving

calories: 304 | fat: 19g | protein: 30g | carbs: 2g | net carbs: 2g | fiber: 0g

Swordfish Skewers with Cherry Tomato

Prep time: 10 minutes | Cook time: 6 to 8 minutes | Serves 4

1 pound (454 g) filleted swordfish

¼ cup avocado oil

2 tablespoons freshly squeezed lemon juice

1 tablespoon minced fresh parsley

2 teaspoons Dijon mustard

Sea salt, freshly ground black pepper, to taste

3 ounces (85 g) cherry tomatoes

1. Cut the fish into 1½-inch chunks, picking out any remaining bones.
2. In a large bowl, whisk together the oil, lemon juice, parsley, and Dijon mustard. Season to taste with salt and pepper. Add the fish and toss to coat the pieces. Cover and marinate the fish chunks in the refrigerator for 30 minutes.
3. Remove the fish from the marinade. Thread the fish and cherry tomatoes on 4 skewers, alternating as you go.
4. Set the air fryer to 400°F (205ºC). Place the skewers in the air fryer basket and cook for 3 minutes. Flip the skewers and cook for 3 to 5 minutes longer, until the fish is cooked through and an instant-read thermometer reads 140°F (60ºC).

Per Serving

calories: 315 | fat: 20g | protein: 29g | carbs: 2g | net carbs: 1g | fiber: 1g

Air Fried Cod Fillet

Prep time: 10 minutes | Cook time: 9 minutes | Serves 4

1 pound (454 g) cod fillets

1½ cups finely ground blanched almond flour

2 teaspoons Old Bay seasoning

½ teaspoon paprika

Sea salt, freshly ground black pepper, to taste

¼ cup sugar-free mayonnaise (homemade, here, or store-bought)

1 large egg, beaten

Avocado oil spray

Elevated Tartar Sauce, for serving

1. Cut the fish into ¾-inch-wide strips.
2. In a shallow bowl, stir together the almond flour, Old Bay seasoning, paprika, and salt and pepper to taste. In another shallow bowl, whisk together the mayonnaise and egg.
3. Dip the cod strips in the egg mixture, then the almond flour, gently pressing with your fingers to help adhere the coating.
4. Place the coated fish on a parchment paper–lined baking sheet and freeze for 30 minutes.

5. Spray the air fryer basket with oil. Set the air fryer to 400°F (205ºC). Place the fish in the basket in a single layer, and spray each piece with oil.
6. Cook for 5 minutes. Flip and spray with more oil. Cook for 4 minutes more, until the internal temperature reaches 140°F (60ºC). Serve with the tartar sauce.

Per Serving

calories: 439 | fat: 33g | protein: 31g | carbs: 9g | net carbs: 4g | fiber: 5g

Cod with Avocado

Prep time: 10 minutes | Cook time: 10 minutes | Serves 2

1 cup shredded cabbage
¼ cup full-fat sour cream
2 tablespoons full-fat mayonnaise
¼ cup chopped pickled jalapeños
2 (3-ounce / (85-g)) cod fillets
1 teaspoon chili powder
1 teaspoon cumin
½ teaspoon paprika
¼ teaspoon garlic powder
1 medium avocado, peeled, pitted, and sliced
½ medium lime

1. In a large bowl, place cabbage, sour cream, mayonnaise, and jalapeños. Mix until fully coated. Let sit for 20 minutes in the refrigerator.
2. Sprinkle cod fillets with chili powder, cumin, paprika, and garlic powder. Place each fillet into the air fryer basket.
3. Adjust the temperature to 370°F (188ºC) and set the timer for 10 minutes.
4. Flip the fillets halfway through the cooking time. When fully cooked, fish should have an internal temperature of at least 145°F (63ºC).
5. To serve, divide slaw mixture into two serving bowls, break cod fillets into pieces and spread over the bowls, and top with avocado. Squeeze lime juice over each bowl. Serve immediately.

Per Serving

calories: 342 | fat: 25g | protein: 16g | carbs: 12g | net carbs: 6g | fiber: 6g

Air Fried Cod Fillets

Prep time: 20 minutes | Cook time: 10 minutes | Serves 2

2 medium-sized cod fillets

½ tablespoon fresh lemon juice

1 ½ tablespoons olive oil

½ tablespoon whole-grain mustard

Sea salt and ground black pepper, to taste

½ cup coconut flour

2 eggs

1. Set your Air Fryer to cook at 355 degrees F (181ºC). Thoroughly combine olive oil and coconut flour in a shallow bowl.
2. In another shallow bowl, whisk the egg. Drizzle each cod fillet with lemon juice and spread with mustard. Then, sprinkle each fillet with salt and ground black pepper.
3. Dip each fish fillet into the whisked egg; now, roll it in the olive oil mixture.
4. Place in a single layer in the Air Fryer cooking basket. Cook for 10 minutes, working in batches, turning once or twice. Serve.

Per Serving

calories: 501 | fat: 35g | protein: 30g | carbs: 32g | net carbs: 31g | fiber: 1g

Cod with Jalapeno

Prep time: 5 minutes | Cook time: 14 minutes | Serves 4

4 cod fillets, boneless

1 jalapeño, minced

1 tablespoon avocado oil

½ teaspoon minced garlic

1. In the shallow bowl, mix minced jalapeño, avocado oil, and minced garlic.
2. Put the cod fillets in the air fryer basket in one layer and top with minced jalapeño mixture.

3. Cook the fish at 365F (185ºC) for 7 minutes per side.

Per Serving

calories: 96 | fat: 2g | protein: 20g | carbs: 2g | net carbs: 1g | fiber: 1g

Air Fried Cod Fillet

Prep time: 10 minutes | Cook time: 7 minutes | Serves 2

12 oz cod fillet
1 teaspoon ground turmeric
1 teaspoon chili flakes
1 tablespoon coconut oil, melted
½ teaspoon salt

1. Mix coconut oil with ground turmeric, chili flakes, and salt.
2. Then mix cod fillet with ground turmeric and put in the air fryer basket.
3. Cook the cod at 385F (196ºC) for 7 minutes.

Per Serving

calories: 199 | fat: 8g | protein: 30g | carbs: 2g | net carbs: 1g | fiber: 1g

Cod with Tomatillos

Prep time: 10 minutes | Cook time: 15 minutes | Serves 4

2 oz tomatillos, chopped
1-pound (454-g) cod fillet, roughly chopped
1 tablespoon avocado oil
1 tablespoon lemon juice
1 teaspoon keto tomato paste

1. Mix avocado oil with lemon juice and tomato paste.
2. Then mix cod fillet with tomato mixture and put in the air fryer.
3. Add lemon juice and tomatillos.

4. Cook the cod at 370F (188ºC) for 15 minutes.

Per Serving

calories: 102 | fat: 2g | protein: 20g | carbs: 2g | net carbs: 1g | fiber: 1g

White Fish with Cauliflower

Prep time: 20 minutes | Cook time: 13 minutes | Serves 4

½ pound (227g) cauliflower florets
½ teaspoon English mustard
2 tablespoons butter, room temperature
½ tablespoon cilantro, minced
2 tablespoons sour cream
2 ½ cups cooked white fish
Salt and freshly cracked black pepper, to taste

1. Boil the cauliflower until tender. Then, purée the cauliflower in your blender. Transfer to a mixing dish.
2. Now, stir in the fish, cilantro, salt, and black pepper.
3. Add the sour cream, English mustard, and butter; mix until everything's well incorporated. Using your hands, shape into patties.
4. Place in the refrigerator for about 2 hours. Cook for 13 minutes at 395 degrees F (202ºC). Serve with some extra English mustard.

Per Serving

calories: 285 | fat: 15g | protein: 31g | carbs: 4g | net carbs: 3g | fiber: 1g

Cheesy Hake Fillet

Prep time: 30 minutes | Cook time: 17 minutes | Serves 4

1 tablespoon avocado oil
1 pound (454 g) hake fillets
1 teaspoon garlic powder
Sea salt and ground white pepper, to taste

2 tablespoons shallots, chopped

1 bell pepper, seeded and chopped

½ cup Cottage cheese

½ cup sour cream

1 egg, well whisked

1 teaspoon yellow mustard

1 tablespoon lime juice

½ cup Swiss cheese, shredded

1. Brush the bottom and sides of a casserole dish with avocado oil. Add the hake fillets to the casserole dish and sprinkle with garlic powder, salt, and pepper.
2. Add the chopped shallots and bell peppers.
3. In a mixing bowl, thoroughly combine the Cottage cheese, sour cream, egg, mustard, and lime juice. Pour the mixture over fish and spread evenly.
4. Cook in the preheated Air Fryer at 370 degrees F (188ºC) for 10 minutes.
5. Top with the Swiss cheese and cook an additional 7 minutes. Let it rest for 10 minutes before slicing and serving. Bon appétit!

Per Serving

calories: 335 | fat: 18g | protein: 34g | carbs: 8g | net carbs: 7g | fiber: 1g

Cheesy Tuna

Prep time: 20 minutes | Cook time: 17 minutes | Serves 4

1 tablespoon butter, melted

1 medium-sized leek, thinly sliced

1 tablespoon chicken stock

1 tablespoon dry white wine

1 pound (454 g) tuna

½ teaspoon red pepper flakes, crushed

Sea salt and ground black pepper, to taste

½ teaspoon dried rosemary

½ teaspoon dried basil

½ teaspoon dried thyme

2 small ripe tomatoes, puréed

1 cup Parmesan cheese, grated

1. Melt ½ tablespoon of butter in a sauté pan over medium-high heat. Now, cook the leek and garlic until tender and aromatic. Add the stock and wine to deglaze the pan.
2. Preheat your Air Fryer to 370 degrees F (188ºC).
3. Grease a casserole dish with the remaining ½ tablespoon of melted butter. Place the fish in the casserole dish. Add the seasonings. Top with the sautéed leek mixture.
4. Add the tomato purée. Cook for 10 minutes in the preheated Air Fryer. Top with grated Parmesan cheese; cook an additional 7 minutes until the crumbs are golden. Bon appétit!

Per Serving

calories: 313 | fat: 15g | protein: 34g | carbs: 8g | net carbs: 7g | fiber: 1g

Grilled Tuna Cake

Prep time: 10 minutes | Cook time: 8 minutes | Serves 4

2 cans canned tuna fish

2 celery stalks, trimmed and finely chopped

1 egg, whisked

½ cup Parmesan cheese, grated

1 teaspoon whole-grain mustard

½ teaspoon sea salt

¼ teaspoon freshly cracked black peppercorns

1 teaspoon paprika

1. Mix all of the above ingredients in the order listed above; mix to combine well and shape into four cakes; chill for 50 minutes.
2. Place on an Air Fryer grill pan. Spritz each cake with a non-stick cooking spray, covering all sides.
3. Grill at 360 degrees F (182ºC) for 5 minutes; then, pause the machine, flip the cakes over and set the timer for another 3 minutes. Serve.

Per Serving

calories: 241 | fat: 11g | protein: 30g | carbs: 2g | net carbs: 1g | fiber: 1g

Tuna Steak

Prep time: 10 minutes | Cook time: 12 minutes | Serves 4

1-pound (454-g) tuna steaks, boneless and cubed

1 tablespoon mustard

1 tablespoon avocado oil

1 tablespoon apple cider vinegar

1. Mix avocado oil with mustard and apple cider vinegar.
2. Then brush tuna steaks with mustard mixture and put in the air fryer basket.
3. Cook the fish at 360F (182ºC) for 6 minutes per side.

Per Serving

calories: 227 | fat: 8g | protein: 34g | carbs: 2g | net carbs: 1g | fiber: 1g

Creamy Tuna Pork Casserole

Prep time: 15 minutes | Cook time: 15 minutes | Serves 4

2 tablespoons salted butter

¼ cup diced white onion

¼ cup chopped white mushrooms

2 stalks celery, finely chopped

½ cup heavy cream

½ cup vegetable broth

2 tablespoons full-fat mayonnaise

¼ teaspoon xanthan gum

½ teaspoon red pepper flakes

2 medium zucchini, spiralized

2 (5-ounce / (142-g)) cans albacore tuna

1 ounce (28 g) pork rinds, finely ground

1. In a large saucepan over medium heat, melt butter. Add onion, mushrooms, and celery and sauté until fragrant, about 3–5 minutes.
2. Pour in heavy cream, vegetable broth, mayonnaise, and xanthan gum. Reduce heat and continue cooking an additional 3 minutes, until the mixture begins to thicken.

3. Add red pepper flakes, zucchini, and tuna. Turn off heat and stir until zucchini noodles are coated.
4. Pour into 4-cup round baking dish. Top with ground pork rinds and cover the top of the dish with foil. Place into the air fryer basket.
5. Adjust the temperature to 370°F (188°C) and set the timer for 15 minutes.
6. When 3 minutes remain, remove the foil to brown the top of the casserole. Serve warm.

Per Serving

calories: 339 | fat: 25g | protein: 20g | carbs: 6g | net carbs: 4g | fiber: 2g

Tuna Avocado Bites

Prep time: 10 minutes | Cook time: 7 minutes | Makes 12 bites

1 (10-ounce / 283-g) can tuna, drained

¼ cup full-fat mayonnaise

1 stalk celery, chopped

1 medium avocado, peeled, pitted, and mashed

½ cup blanched finely ground almond flour, divided

2 teaspoons coconut oil

1. In a large bowl, mix tuna, mayonnaise, celery, and mashed avocado. Form the mixture into balls.
2. Roll balls in almond flour and spritz with coconut oil. Place balls into the air fryer basket.
3. Adjust the temperature to 400°F (205°C) and set the timer for 7 minutes.
4. Gently turn tuna bites after 5 minutes. Serve warm.

Per Serving

calories: 323 | fat: 25g | protein: 17g | carbs: 6g | net carbs: 2g | fiber: 4g

Rockfish with Avocado Cream

Prep time: 15 minutes | Cook time: 9 minutes | Serves 4

For the Fish Fillets:

1½ tablespoons balsamic vinegar

½ cup vegetable broth

⅓ teaspoon shallot powder

1 tablespoon coconut aminos

4 Rockfish fillets

1 teaspoon ground black pepper

1½ tablespoons olive oil

Fine sea salt, to taste

⅓ teaspoon garlic powder

For the Avocado Cream:

2 tablespoons Greek-style yogurt

1 clove garlic, peeled and minced

1 teaspoon ground black pepper

½ tablespoon olive oil

⅓ cup vegetable broth

1 avocado

½ teaspoon lime juice

⅓ teaspoon fine sea salt

1. In a bowl, wash and pat the fillets dry using some paper towels. Add all the seasonings. In another bowl, stir in the remaining ingredients for the fish fillets.
2. Add the seasoned fish fillets; cover and let the fillets marinate in your refrigerator at least 3 hours.
3. Then, set your Air Fryer to cook at 325 degrees F (163ºC). Cook marinated rockfish fillets in the air fryer grill basket for 9 minutes.
4. In the meantime, prepare the avocado sauce by mixing all the ingredients with an immersion blender or regular blender. Serve the rockfish fillets topped with the avocado sauce. Enjoy!

Per Serving

calories: 347 | fat: 25g | protein: 3g | carbs: 7g | net carbs: 4g | fiber: 3g

Whitefish Fillet with Green Bean

Prep time: 1 hour 20 minutes | Cook time: 15 minutes | Serves 4

1 pound (454 g) whitefish fillets, minced

½ pound (227g) green beans, finely chopped

½ cup scallions, chopped

1 chili pepper, seeded and minced

1 tablespoon red curry paste

1 tablespoon fish sauce

2 tablespoons apple cider vinegar

1 teaspoon water

Sea salt flakes, to taste

½ teaspoon cracked black peppercorns

2 tablespoons butter, at room temperature

½ teaspoon lemon

1. Add all ingredients in the order listed above to the mixing dish. Mix to combine well using a spatula or your hands.
2. Form into small cakes and chill for 1 hour. Place a piece of aluminum foil over the cooking basket. Place the cakes on foil.
3. Cook at 390 degrees F (199ºC) for 10 minutes; pause the machine, flip each fish cake over and air-fry for additional 5 minutes. Mound a cucumber relish onto the plates; add the fish cakes and serve warm.

Per Serving

calories: 231 | fat: 12g | protein: 23g | carbs: 6g | net carbs: 4g | fiber: 2g

Baked Monkfish

Prep time: 20 minutes | Cook time: 12 minutes | Serves 2

2 teaspoons olive oil

1 cup celery, sliced

2 bell peppers, sliced

1 teaspoon dried thyme

½ teaspoon dried marjoram

½ teaspoon dried rosemary

2 monkfish fillets

1 tablespoon coconut aminos

2 tablespoons lime juice

Coarse salt and ground black pepper, to taste

1 teaspoon cayenne pepper

½ cup Kalamata olives, pitted and sliced

1. In a nonstick skillet, heat the olive oil for 1 minute. Once hot, sauté the celery and peppers until tender, about 4 minutes. Sprinkle with thyme, marjoram, and rosemary and set aside.
2. Toss the fish fillets with the coconut aminos, lime juice, salt, black pepper, and cayenne pepper. Place the fish fillets in a lightly greased cooking basket and bake at 390 degrees F (199ºC) for 8 minutes.
3. Turn them over, add the olives, and cook an additional 4 minutes. Serve with the sautéed vegetables on the side. Bon appétit!

Per Serving

calories: 292 | fat: 19g | protein: 22g | carbs: 9g | net carbs: 6g | fiber: 3g

Cheesy Flounder Cutlets

Prep time: 15 minutes | Cook time: 10 minutes | Serves 2

1 egg

1 cup Pecorino Romano cheese, grated

Sea salt and white pepper, to taste

½ teaspoon cayenne pepper

1 teaspoon dried parsley flakes

2 flounder fillets

1. To make a breading station, whisk the egg until frothy.
2. In another bowl, mix Pecorino Romano cheese, and spices.
3. Dip the fish in the egg mixture and turn to coat evenly; then, dredge in the cracker crumb mixture, turning a couple of times to coat evenly.
4. Cook in the preheated Air Fryer at 390 degrees F (199ºC) for 5 minutes; turn them over and cook another 5 minutes. Enjoy!

Per Serving

calories: 425 | fat: 26g | protein: 37g | carbs: 7g | net carbs: 7g | fiber: 0g

Roast Swordfish Steak

Prep time: 30 minutes | Cook time: 20 minutes | Serves 3

3 bell peppers

3 swordfish steaks

1 tablespoon butter, melted

2 garlic cloves, minced

Sea salt and freshly ground black pepper, to taste

½ teaspoon cayenne pepper

½ teaspoon ginger powder

1. Start by preheating your Air Fryer to 400 degrees F (205ºC). Brush the Air Fryer basket lightly with cooking oil.
2. Then, roast the bell peppers for 5 minutes. Give the peppers a half turn; place them back in the cooking basket and roast for another 5 minutes.
3. Turn them one more time and roast until the skin is charred and soft or 5 more minutes. Peel the peppers and set aside.
4. Then, add the swordfish steaks to the lightly greased cooking basket and cook at 400 degrees F (205ºC) for 10 minutes.
5. Meanwhile, melt the butter in a small saucepan. Cook the garlic until fragrant and add the salt, pepper, cayenne pepper, and ginger powder. Cook until everything is thoroughly heated.
6. Plate the peeled peppers and the roasted swordfish; spoon the sauce over them and serve warm.

Per Serving

calories: 460 | fat: 17g | protein: 66g | carbs: 5g | net carbs: 4g | fiber: 1g

Snapper with Shallot and Tomato

Prep time: 20 minutes | Cook time: 15 minutes | Serves 2

2 snapper fillets

1 shallot, peeled and sliced

2 garlic cloves, halved

1 bell pepper, sliced

1 small-sized serrano pepper, sliced

1 tomato, sliced

1 tablespoon olive oil

¼ teaspoon freshly ground black pepper

½ teaspoon paprika

Sea salt, to taste

2 bay leaves

1. Place two parchment sheets on a working surface. Place the fish in the center of one side of the parchment paper.
2. Top with the shallot, garlic, peppers, and tomato. Drizzle olive oil over the fish and vegetables. Season with black pepper, paprika, and salt. Add the bay leaves.
3. Fold over the other half of the parchment. Now, fold the paper around the edges tightly and create a half moon shape, sealing the fish inside.
4. Cook in the preheated Air Fryer at 390 degrees F (199ºC) for 15 minutes. Serve warm.

Per Serving

calories: 329 | fat: 9g | protein: 47g | carbs: 13g | net carbs: 12g | fiber: 1g

Lemony Salmon Steak

Prep time: 20 minutes | Cook time: 12 minutes | Serves 2

2 salmon steaks

Coarse sea salt, to taste

¼ teaspoon freshly ground black pepper, or more to taste

1 tablespoon sesame oil

Zest of 1 lemon

1 tablespoon fresh lemon juice

1 teaspoon garlic, minced

½ teaspoon smoked cayenne pepper

½ teaspoon dried dill

1. Preheat your Air Fryer to 380 degrees F (193ºC). Pat dry the salmon steaks with a kitchen towel.
2. In a ceramic dish, combine the remaining ingredients until everything is well whisked.
3. Add the salmon steaks to the ceramic dish and let them sit in the refrigerator for 1 hour. Now, place the salmon steaks in the cooking basket. Reserve the marinade.
4. Cook for 12 minutes, flipping halfway through the cooking time.

5. Meanwhile, cook the marinade in a small sauté pan over a moderate flame. Cook until the sauce has thickened.
6. Pour the sauce over the steaks and serve. Bon appétit!

Per Serving

calories: 476 | fat: 16g | protein: 47g | carbs: 3g | net carbs: 2g | fiber: 1g

Air Fried Salmon

Prep time: 50 minutes | Cook time: 10 minutes | Serves 4

1½ pounds (680g) salmon steak

½ teaspoon grated lemon zest

Freshly cracked mixed peppercorns, to taste

⅓ cup lemon juice

Fresh chopped chives, for garnish

½ cup dry white wine

½ teaspoon fresh cilantro, chopped

Fine sea salt, to taste

1. To prepare the marinade, place all ingredients, except for salmon steak and chives, in a deep pan. Bring to a boil over medium-high flame until it has reduced by half. Allow it to cool down.
2. After that, allow salmon steak to marinate in the refrigerator approximately 40 minutes. Discard the marinade and transfer the fish steak to the preheated Air Fryer.
3. Air-fry at 400 degrees F (205ºC) for 9 to10 minutes. To finish, brush hot fish steaks with the reserved marinade, garnish with fresh chopped chives, and serve right away!

Per Serving

calories: 304 | fat: 15g | protein: 38g | carbs: 2g | net carbs: 1g | fiber: 1g

Savory Salmon Fillet

Prep time: 10 minutes | Cook time: 8 minutes | Serves 2

10 oz salmon fillet
½ teaspoon ground coriander
1 teaspoon ground cumin
1 teaspoon dried basil
1 tablespoon avocado oil

1. In the shallow bowl, mix ground coriander, ground cumin, and dried basil.
2. Then coat the salmon fillet in the spices and sprinkle with avocado oil.
3. Put the fish in the air fryer basket and cook at 395F (202ºC) for 4 minutes per side.

Per Serving

calories: 201 | fat: 9g | protein: 28g | carbs: 1g | net carbs: 0g | fiber: 1g

Salmon with Provolone Cheese

Prep time: 5 minutes | Cook time: 15 minutes | Serves 4

1-pound (454-g) salmon fillet, chopped
2 oz Provolone, grated
1 teaspoon avocado oil
¼ teaspoon ground paprika

1. Sprinkle the salmon fillets with avocado oil and put in the air fryer.
2. Then sprinkle the fish with ground paprika and top with Provolone cheese.
3. Cook the fish at 360F (182ºC) for 15 minutes.

Per Serving

calories: 202 | fat: 10g | protein: 26g | carbs: 1g | net carbs: 0g | fiber: 1g

Salmon with Endives

Prep time: 5 minutes | Cook time: 20 minutes | Serves 4

2 endives, shredded

1-pound (454-g) salmon fillet, chopped

1 tablespoon ghee

1 teaspoon ground coriander

¼ cup coconut cream

1. Put all ingredients in the air fryer and shake gently.
2. Close the lid and cook the meal ay 360F (182ºC) for 20 minutes. Shake the fish every 5 minutes.

Per Serving

calories: 223 | fat: 13g | protein: 23g | carbs: 3g | net carbs: 1g | fiber: 2g

Salmon Fritters with Zucchini

Prep time: 15 minutes | Cook time: 12 minutes | Serves 4

2 tablespoons almond flour

1 zucchini, grated

1 egg, beaten

6 oz salmon fillet, diced

1 teaspoon avocado oil

½ teaspoon ground black pepper

1. Mix almond flour with zucchini, egg, salmon, and ground black pepper.
2. Then make the fritters from the salmon mixture.
3. Sprinkle the air fryer basket with avocado oil and put the fritters inside.
4. Cook the fritters at 375F (190ºC) for 6 minutes per side.

Per Serving

calories: 103 | fat: 5g | protein: 11g | carbs: 3g | net carbs: 2g | fiber: 1g

Air Fried Salmon Fillet

Prep time: 15 minutes | Cook time: 15 minutes | Serves 4

1-pound (454-g) salmon fillet

4 kalamata olives, sliced

1 teaspoon avocado oil

1 teaspoon Italian seasonings

2 oz Mozzarella, shredded

1. Make the cut in the salmon in the shape of the pocket.
2. The fill the salmon cut with olives and Mozzarella.
3. Secure the cut with the help of the toothpick and sprinkle the salmon with Italian seasonings and avocado oil.
4. Cook the salmon in the air fryer basket and cook it at 380F (193ºC) for 15 minutes.

Per Serving

calories: 200 | fat: 10g | protein: 26g | carbs: 2g | net carbs: 1g | fiber: 1g

Tasty Salmon

Prep time: 15 minutes | Cook time: 8 minutes | Serves 4

2-pound (907-g) salmon fillet

¼ cup coconut shred

2 eggs, beaten

1 teaspoon coconut oil

1 teaspoon Italian seasonings

1. Cut the salmon fillet into servings.
2. Then sprinkle the fish with Italian seasonings and dip in the eggs.
3. After this, coat every salmon fillet in coconut shred and put it in the air fryer.
4. Cook the fish at 375F (190ºC) for 4 minutes per side.

Per Serving

calories: 395 | fat: 22g | protein: 47g | carbs: 2g | net carbs: 1g | fiber: 1g

Salmon with Cauliflower

Prep time: 10 minutes | Cook time: 25 minutes | Serves 4

1-pound (454-g) salmon fillet, diced
1 cup cauliflower, shredded
1 tablespoon dried cilantro
1 tablespoon coconut oil, melted
1 teaspoon ground turmeric
¼ cup coconut cream

1. Mix salmon with cauliflower, dried cilantro, ground turmeric, coconut cream, and coconut oil.
2. Transfer the salmon mixture in the air fryer and cook the meal at 350F (180ºC) for 25 minutes. Stir the meal every 5 minutes to avoid the burning.

Per Serving

calories: 222 | fat: 14g | protein: 23g | carbs: 3g | net carbs: 2g | fiber: 1g

Lemony Salmon

Prep time: 10 minutes | Cook time: 12 minutes | Serves 2

2 (4-ounce / (113 g)) salmon fillets, skin removed
2 tablespoons unsalted butter, melted
½ teaspoon garlic powder
1 medium lemon
½ teaspoon dried dill

1. Place each fillet on a 5-inch × 5-inch square of aluminum foil. Drizzle with butter and sprinkle with garlic powder.
2. Zest half of the lemon and sprinkle zest over salmon. Slice other half of the lemon and lay two slices on each piece of salmon. Sprinkle dill over salmon.
3. Gather and fold foil at the top and sides to fully close packets. Place foil packets into the air fryer basket.
4. Adjust the temperature to 400°F (205ºC) and set the timer for 12 minutes.

5. Salmon will be easily flaked and have an internal temperature of at least 145°F (63ºC) when fully cooked. Serve immediately.

Per Serving

calories: 252 | fat: 16g | protein: 20g | carbs: 2g | net carbs: 1g | fiber: 1g

Crispy Salmon Patties

Prep time: 10 minutes | Cook time: 8 minutes | Serves 2

2 (5-ounce / (142 g)) pouches cooked pink salmon

1 large egg

¼ cup ground pork rinds

2 tablespoons full-fat mayonnaise

2 teaspoons sriracha

1 teaspoon chili powder

1. Mix all ingredients in a large bowl and form into four patties. Place patties into the air fryer basket.
2. Adjust the temperature to 400°F (205ºC) and set the timer for 8 minutes.
3. Carefully flip each patty halfway through the cooking time. Patties will be crispy on the outside when fully cooked.

Per Serving

calories: 319 | fat: 19g | protein: 34g | carbs: 2g | net carbs: 1g | fiber: 1g

Air Fried Salmon

Prep time: 5 minutes | Cook time: 12 minutes | Serves 2

¼ cup pesto

¼ cup sliced almonds, roughly chopped

2 (1½ -inch-thick) salmon fillets (about 4 ounces each/ 113 g)

2 tablespoons unsalted butter, melted

1. In a small bowl, mix pesto and almonds. Set aside.
2. Place fillets into a 6 -inch round baking dish.

3. Brush each fillet with butter and place half of the pesto mixture on the top of each fillet. Place dish into the air fryer basket.
4. Adjust the temperature to 390°F (199ºC) and set the timer for 12 minutes.
5. Salmon will easily flake when fully cooked and reach an internal temperature of at least 145°F (63ºC). Serve warm.

Per Serving

calories: 433 | fat: 34g | protein: 23g | carbs: 6g | net carbs: 4g | fiber: 2g

Air Fried Catfish

Prep time: 10 minutes | Cook time: 12 minutes | Serves 4

2-pound (907-g) catfish fillet

½ cup almond flour

2 eggs, beaten

1 teaspoon salt

1 teaspoon avocado oil

1. Sprinkle the catfish fillet with salt and dip in the eggs.
2. Then coat the fish in the almond flour and put in the air fryer basket. Sprinkle the fish with avocado oil.
3. Cook the fish for 6 minutes per side at 380F (193ºC).

Per Serving

calories: 423 | fat: 26g | protein: 41g | carbs: 3g | net carbs: 1g | fiber: 2g

Tilapia with Pecan

Prep time: 20 minutes | Cook time: 16 minutes | Serves 5

2 tablespoons ground flaxseeds

1 teaspoon paprika

Sea salt and white pepper, to taste

1 teaspoon garlic paste

2 tablespoons extra-virgin olive oil

½ cup pecans, ground

5 tilapia fillets, slice into halves

1. Combine the ground flaxseeds, paprika, salt, white pepper, garlic paste, olive oil, and ground pecans in a Ziploc bag. Add the fish fillets and shake to coat well.
2. Spritz the Air Fryer basket with cooking spray. Cook in the preheated Air Fryer at 400 degrees F (205ºC) for 10 minutes; turn them over and cook for 6 minutes more. Work in batches.
3. Serve with lemon wedges, if desired. Enjoy!

Per Serving

calories: 264 | fat: 17g | protein: 6g | carbs: 4g | net carbs: 2g | fiber: 2g

Easy Tilapia Fillet

Prep time: 5 minutes | Cook time: 15 minutes | Serves 4

4 tilapia fillets, boneless

2 tablespoons balsamic vinegar

1 teaspoon avocado oil

1 teaspoon dried basil

1. Sprinkle the tilapia fillets with balsamic vinegar, avocado oil, and dried basil.
2. Then put the fillets in the air fryer basket and cook at 365F (185ºC) for 15 minutes.

Per Serving

calories: 96 | fat: 1g | protein: 21g | carbs: 1g | net carbs: 0g | fiber: 1g

Savory Tilapia

Prep time: 5 minutes | Cook time: 20 minutes | Serves 4

4 tilapia fillets, boneless

1 teaspoon chili flakes

1 teaspoon dried oregano

1 tablespoon avocado oil

1 teaspoon mustard

1. Rub the tilapia fillets with chili flakes, dried oregano, avocado oil, and mustard and put in the air fryer.
2. Cook it for 10 minutes per side at 360F (182ºC).

Per Serving

calories: 103 | fat: 1g | protein: 21g | carbs: 1g | net carbs: 0g | fiber: 1g

Sweet Tilapia Fillets

Prep time: 5 minutes | Cook time: 14 minutes | Serves 4

2 tablespoons erythritol

1 tablespoon apple cider vinegar

4 tilapia fillets, boneless

1 teaspoon olive oil

1. Mix apple cider vinegar with olive oil and erythritol.
2. Then rub the tilapia fillets with the sweet mixture and put in the air fryer basket in one layer.
3. Cook the fish at 360F (182ºC) for 7 minutes per side.

Per Serving

calories: 101 | fat: 2g | protein: 20g | carbs: 0g | net carbs: 0g | fiber: 0g

Air Fried Tilapia

Prep time: 15 minutes | Cook time: 9 minutes | Serves 4

1-pound (454-g) tilapia fillet

½ cup coconut flour

2 eggs, beaten

½ teaspoon ground paprika

1 teaspoon dried oregano

1 teaspoon avocado oil

1. Cut the tilapia fillets into fingers and sprinkle with ground paprika and dried oregano.
2. Then dip the tilapia fingers in eggs and coat in the coconut flour.
3. Sprinkle fish fingers with avocado oil and cook in the air fryer at 370F (188ºC) for 9 minutes.

Per Serving

calories: 188 | fat: 5g | protein: 26g | carbs: 9g | net carbs: 4g | fiber: 5g

Quick Tilapia

Prep time: 15 minutes | Cook time: 10 minutes | Serves 4

2-pound (907-g) tilapia fillet

1 teaspoon fennel seeds

1 tablespoon avocado oil

½ teaspoon lime zest, grated

1 tablespoon coconut aminos

1. In the shallow bowl, mix fennel seeds with avocado oil, lime zest, and coconut aminos.
2. Then brush the tilapia fillet with fennel seeds and put in the air fryer.
3. Cook the fish at 380F (193ºC) for 10 minutes.

Per Serving

calories: 194 | fat: 2g | protein: 42g | carbs: 1g | net carbs: 0g | fiber: 1g

Creamy Haddock

Prep time: 10 minutes | Cook time: 8 minutes | Serves 4

1-pound (454-g) haddock fillet

1 teaspoon cayenne pepper

1 teaspoon salt

1 teaspoon coconut oil

½ cup heavy cream

1. Grease the baking pan with coconut oil.
2. Then put haddock fillet inside and sprinkle it with cayenne pepper, salt, and heavy cream.
3. Put the baking pan in the air fryer basket and cook at 375F (190ºC) for 8 minutes.

Per Serving

calories: 190 | fat: 7g | protein: 28g | carbs: 2g | net carbs: 1g | fiber: 1g

Mackerel with Spinach

Prep time: 15 minutes | Cook time: 20 minutes | Serves 5

1-pound (454 g) mackerel, trimmed

1 bell pepper, chopped

½ cup spinach, chopped

1 tablespoon avocado oil

1 teaspoon ground black pepper

1 teaspoon keto tomato paste

1. In the mixing bowl, mix bell pepper with spinach, ground black pepper, and tomato paste.
2. Fill the mackerel with spinach mixture.
3. Then brush the fish with avocado oil and put it in the air fryer.
4. Cook the fish at 365F (185ºC) for 20 minutes.

Per Serving

calories: 252 | fat: 16g | protein: 22g | carbs: 2g | net carbs: 1g | fiber: 1g

Air Fried Mackerel Fillet

Prep time: 10 minutes | Cook time: 7 minutes | Serves 2

12 oz mackerel fillet

2 oz Parmesan, grated

1 teaspoon ground coriander

1 tablespoon olive oil

1. Sprinkle the mackerel fillet with olive oil and put it in the air fryer basket.
2. Top the fish with ground coriander and Parmesan.
3. Cook the fish at 390F (199ºC) for 7 minutes.

Per Serving

calories: 597 | fat: 43g | protein: 50g | carbs: 1g | net carbs: 1g | fiber: 0g

Creamy Mackerel

Prep time: 10 minutes | Cook time: 6 minutes | Serves 4

2-pound (907-g) mackerel fillet

1 cup coconut cream

1 teaspoon ground coriander

1 teaspoon cumin seeds

1 garlic clove, peeled, chopped

1. Chop the mackerel roughly and sprinkle it with coconut cream, ground coriander, cumin seeds, and garlic.
2. Then put the fish in the air fryer and cook at 400F (205ºC) for 6 minutes.

Per Serving

calories: 735 | fat: 54g | protein: 55g | carbs: 4g | net carbs: 2g | fiber: 2g

Easy Sardines

Prep time: 15 minutes | Cook time: 10 minutes | Serves 5

12 oz sardines, trimmed, cleaned

1 cup coconut flour

1 tablespoon coconut oil

1 teaspoon salt

1. Sprinkle the sardines with salt and coat in the coconut flour.
2. Then grease the air fryer basket with coconut oil and put the sardines inside.

3. Cook them at 385F (196ºC) for 10 minutes.

Per Serving

calories: 165 | fat: 10g | protein: 17g | carbs: 1g | net carbs: 1g | fiber: 0g

Bacon Halibut Steak

Prep time: 15 minutes | Cook time: 10 minutes | Serves 4

24 oz halibut steaks (6 oz each fillet)

1 teaspoon avocado oil

1 teaspoon ground black pepper

4 oz bacon, sliced

1. Sprinkle the halibut steaks with avocado oil and ground black pepper.
2. Then wrap the fish in the bacon slices and put in the air fryer.
3. Cook the fish at 390F (199ºC) for 5 minutes per side.

Per Serving

calories: 266 | fat: 14g | protein: 33g | carbs: 2g | net carbs: 1g | fiber: 1g

Shrimp with Romaine

Prep time: 10 minutes | Cook time: 4 to 6 minutes | Serves 4

12 ounces (340 g) fresh large shrimp, peeled and deveined

1 tablespoon plus 1 teaspoon freshly squeezed lemon juice, divided

4 tablespoons olive oil or avocado oil, divided

2 garlic cloves, minced, divided

¼ teaspoon sea salt, plus additional to season the marinade

¼ teaspoon freshly ground black pepper, plus additional to season the marinade

$1/3$ cup sugar-free mayonnaise (homemade, here, or store-bought)

2 tablespoons freshly grated Parmesan cheese

1 teaspoon Dijon mustard

1 tinned anchovy, mashed

12 ounces (340 g) romaine hearts, torn

1. Place the shrimp in a large bowl. Add 1 tablespoon of lemon juice, 1 tablespoon of olive oil, and 1 minced garlic clove. Season with salt and pepper. Toss well and refrigerate for 15 minutes.
2. While the shrimp marinates, make the dressing: In a blender, combine the mayonnaise, Parmesan cheese, Dijon mustard, the remaining 1 teaspoon of lemon juice, the anchovy, the remaining minced garlic clove, ¼ teaspoon of salt, and ¼ teaspoon of pepper. Process until smooth. With the blender running, slowly stream in the remaining 3 tablespoons of oil. Transfer the mixture to a jar; seal and refrigerate until ready to serve.
3. Remove the shrimp from its marinade and place it in the air fryer basket in a single layer. Set the air fryer to 400°F (205ºC) and cook for 2 minutes. Flip the shrimp and cook for 2 to 4 minutes more, until the flesh turns opaque.
4. Place the romaine in a large bowl and toss with the desired amount of dressing. Top with the shrimp and serve immediately.

Per Serving

calories: 329 | fat: 30g | protein: 16g | carbs: 4g | net carbs: 2g | fiber: 2g

Air Fried Shrimp

Prep time: 15 minutes | Cook time: 17 minutes | Serves 4

¾ cup unsweetened shredded coconut

¾ cup coconut flour

1 teaspoon garlic powder

¼ teaspoon cayenne pepper

Sea salt, freshly ground black pepper, to taste

2 large eggs

1 pound (454 g) fresh extra-large or jumbo shrimp, peeled and deveined

Avocado oil spray

1. In a medium bowl, combine the shredded coconut, coconut flour, garlic powder, and cayenne pepper. Season to taste with salt and pepper.
2. In a small bowl, beat the eggs.
3. Pat the shrimp dry with paper towels. Dip each shrimp in the eggs and then the coconut mixture. Gently press the coating to the shrimp to help it adhere.

4. Set the air fryer to 400°F (205ºC). Spray the shrimp with oil and place them in a single layer in the air fryer basket, working in batches if necessary.
5. Cook the shrimp for 9 minutes, then flip and spray them with more oil. Cook for 8 minutes more, until the center of the shrimp is opaque and cooked through.

Per Serving

calories: 362 | fat: 17g | protein: 35g | carbs: 20g | net carbs: 9g | fiber: 11g

Savory Shrimp

Prep time: 5 minutes | Cook time: 8 to 10 minutes | Serves 4

1 pound (454 g) fresh large shrimp, peeled and deveined

1 tablespoon avocado oil

2 teaspoons minced garlic, divided

½ teaspoon red pepper flakes

Sea salt, freshly ground black pepper, to taste

2 tablespoons unsalted butter, melted

2 tablespoons chopped fresh parsley

1. Place the shrimp in a large bowl and toss with the avocado oil, 1 teaspoon of minced garlic, and red pepper flakes. Season with salt and pepper.
2. Set the air fryer to 350°F (180ºC). Arrange the shrimp in a single layer in the air fryer basket, working in batches if necessary. Cook for 6 minutes. Flip the shrimp and cook for 2 to 4 minutes more, until the internal temperature of the shrimp reaches 120°F (49ºC). (The time it takes to cook will depend on the size of the shrimp.)
3. While the shrimp are cooking, melt the butter in a small saucepan over medium heat and stir in the remaining 1 teaspoon of garlic.
4. Transfer the cooked shrimp to a large bowl, add the garlic butter, and toss well. Top with the parsley and serve warm.

Per Serving

calories: 220 | fat: 11g | protein: 28g | carbs: 2g | net carbs: 1g | fiber: 1g

Buttery Scallops

Prep time: 5 minutes | Cook time: 15 minutes | Serves 4

1 pound (454 g) large sea scallops

Sea salt, freshly ground black pepper, to taste

Avocado oil spray

¼ cup (4 tablespoons) unsalted butter

1 tablespoon freshly squeezed lemon juice

1 teaspoon minced garlic

¼ teaspoon red pepper flakes

1. If your scallops still have the adductor muscles attached, remove them. Pat the scallops dry with a paper towel.
2. Season the scallops with salt and pepper, then place them on a plate and refrigerate for 15 minutes.
3. Spray the air fryer basket with oil, and arrange the scallops in a single layer. Spray the top of the scallops with oil.
4. Set the air fryer to 350°F (180ºC) and cook for 6 minutes. Flip the scallops and cook for 6 minutes more, until an instant-read thermometer reads 145° F (63ºC).
5. While the scallops cook, place the butter, lemon juice, garlic, and red pepper flakes in a small ramekin.
6. When the scallops have finished cooking, remove them from the air fryer. Place the ramekin in the air fryer and cook until the butter melts, about 3 minutes. Stir.
7. Toss the scallops with the warm butter and serve.

Per Serving

calories: 203 | fat: 12g | protein: 19g | carbs: 3g | net carbs: 3g | fiber: 0g

Crab Cake

Prep time: 10 minutes | Cook time: 14 minutes | Serves 4

Avocado oil spray

$1/3$ cup red onion, diced

¼ cup red bell pepper, diced

8 ounces (227 g) lump crab meat, picked over for shells

3 tablespoons finely ground blanched almond flour

1 large egg, beaten

1 tablespoon sugar-free mayonnaise (homemade, here, or store-bought)

2 teaspoons Dijon mustard

⅛ teaspoon cayenne pepper

Sea salt, freshly ground black pepper, to taste

[Elevated Tartar Sauce](#), for serving

Lemon wedges, for serving

1. Spray an air fryer–friendly baking pan with oil. Put the onion and red bell pepper in the pan and give them a quick spray with oil. Place the pan in the air fryer basket. Set the air fryer to 400°F (205ºC) and cook the vegetables for 7 minutes, until tender.
2. Transfer the vegetables to a large bowl. Add the crab meat, almond flour, egg, mayonnaise, mustard, and cayenne pepper and season with salt and pepper. Stir until the mixture is well combined.
3. Form the mixture into four 1-inch-thick cakes. Cover with plastic wrap and refrigerate for 1 hour.
4. Place the crab cakes in a single layer in the air fryer basket and spray them with oil.
5. Cook for 4 minutes. Flip the crab cakes and spray with more oil. Cook for 3 minutes more, until the internal temperature of the crab cakes reaches 155°F (68ºC).
6. Serve with tartar sauce and a squeeze of fresh lemon juice.

Per Serving

calories: 121 | fat: 8g | protein: 11g | carbs: 3g | net carbs: 2g | fiber: 1g

Easy Shrimp

Prep time: 5 minutes | Cook time: 6 minutes | Serves 2

8 ounces (227 g) medium shelled and deveined shrimp

2 tablespoons salted butter, melted

1 teaspoon paprika

½ teaspoon garlic powder

¼ teaspoon onion powder

½ teaspoon Old Bay seasoning

1. Toss all ingredients together in a large bowl. Place shrimp into the air fryer basket.
2. Adjust the temperature to 400°F (205ºC) and set the timer for 6 minutes.
3. Turn the shrimp halfway through the cooking time to ensure even cooking. Serve immediately.

Per Serving

calories: 192 | fat: 11g | protein: 17g | carbs: 3g | net carbs: 2g | fiber: 1g

Air Fried Shrimp

Prep time: 10 minutes | Cook time: 7 minutes | Serves 4

1 pound (454 g) medium shelled and deveined shrimp

2 tablespoons salted butter, melted

½ teaspoon Old Bay seasoning

¼ teaspoon garlic powder

2 tablespoons sriracha

¼ teaspoon powdered erythritol

¼ cup full-fat mayonnaise

⅛ teaspoon ground black pepper

1. In a large bowl, toss shrimp in butter, Old Bay seasoning, and garlic powder. Place shrimp into the air fryer basket.
2. Adjust the temperature to 400°F (205ºC) and set the timer for 7 minutes.
3. Flip the shrimp halfway through the cooking time. Shrimp will be bright pink when fully cooked.
4. In another large bowl, mix sriracha, powdered erythritol, mayonnaise, and pepper. Toss shrimp in the spicy mixture and serve immediately.

Per Serving

calories: 143 | fat: 6g | protein: 16g | carbs: 3g | net carbs: 3g | fiber: 0g

Golden Shrimp

Prep time: 20 minutes | Cook time: 7 minutes | Serves 4

2 egg whites

½ cup coconut flour

1 cup Parmigiano-Reggiano, grated

½ teaspoon celery seeds

½ teaspoon porcini powder

½ teaspoon onion powder

1 teaspoon garlic powder

½ teaspoon dried rosemary

½ teaspoon sea salt

½ teaspoon ground black pepper

1½ pounds (680g) shrimp, deveined

1. Whisk the egg with coconut flour and Parmigiano-Reggiano. Add in seasonings and mix to combine well.
2. Dip your shrimp in the batter. Roll until they are covered on all sides.
3. Cook in the preheated Air Fryer at 390 degrees F (199ºC) for 5 to 7 minutes or until golden brown. Work in batches. Serve with lemon wedges if desired.

Per Serving

calories: 300 | fat: 11g | protein: 44g | carbs: 7g | net carbs: 6g | fiber: 1g

Cheesy Shrimp

Prep time: 15 minutes | Cook time: 5 minutes | Serves 4

14 oz shrimps, peeled

1 egg, beaten

½ cup of coconut milk

1 cup Cheddar cheese, shredded

½ teaspoon coconut oil

1 teaspoon ground coriander

1. In the mixing bowl, mix shrimps with egg, coconut milk, Cheddar cheese, coconut oil, and ground coriander.
2. Then put the mixture in the baking ramekins and put in the air fryer.
3. Cook the shrimps at 400F (205ºC) for 5 minutes.

Per Serving

calories: 321 | fat: 19g | protein: 32g | carbs: 4g | net carbs: 3g | fiber: 1g

Shrimp with Swiss Chard

Prep time: 10 minutes | Cook time: 10 minutes | Serves 4

1-pound (454-g) shrimp, peeled and deveined
½ teaspoon smoked paprika
½ cup Swiss chard, chopped
2 tablespoons apple cider vinegar
1 tablespoon coconut oil
¼ cup heavy cream

1. Mix shrimps with smoked paprika and apple cider vinegar.
2. Put the shrimps in the air fryer and add coconut oil.
3. Cook the shrimps at 350F (180ºC) for 10 minutes.
4. Then mix cooked shrimps with remaining ingredients and carefully mix.

Per Serving
calories: 193 | fat: 8g | protein: 26g | carbs: 2g | net carbs: 1g | fiber: 1g

Cheesy Crab Patties

Prep time: 20 minutes | Cook time: 14 minutes | Serves 3

2 eggs, beaten
1 shallot, chopped
2 garlic cloves, crushed
1 tablespoon olive oil
1 teaspoon yellow mustard
1 teaspoon fresh cilantro, chopped
10 ounces (283 g) crab meat
1 teaspoon smoked paprika
½ teaspoon ground black pepper
Sea salt, to taste
¾ cup Parmesan cheese

1. In a mixing bowl, thoroughly combine the eggs, shallot, garlic, olive oil, mustard, cilantro, crab meat, paprika, black pepper, and salt. Mix until well combined.

2. Shape the mixture into 6 patties. Roll the crab patties over grated Parmesan cheese, coating well on all sides. Place in your refrigerator for 2 hours.
3. Spritz the crab patties with cooking oil on both sides. Cook in the preheated Air Fryer at 360 degrees F (182ºC) for 14 minutes. Serve on dinner rolls if desired. Bon appétit!

Per Serving

calories: 279 | fat: 15g | protein: 28g | carbs: 6g | net carbs: 5g | fiber: 1g

Air Fried Crab Bun

Prep time: 15 minutes | Cook time: 20 minutes | Serves 2

5 oz crab meat, chopped

2 eggs, beaten

2 tablespoons coconut flour

¼ teaspoon baking powder

½ teaspoon coconut aminos

½ teaspoon ground black pepper

1 tablespoon coconut oil, softened

1. In the mixing bowl, mix crab meat with eggs, coconut flour, baking powder, coconut aminos, ground black pepper, and coconut oil.
2. Knead the smooth dough and cut it into pieces.
3. Make the buns from the crab mixture and put them in the air fryer basket.
4. Cook the crab buns at 365F (185ºC) for 20 minutes.

Per Serving

calories: 217 | fat: 13g | protein: 15g | carbs: 7g | net carbs: 4g | fiber: 3g

Quick Shrimp Skewers

Prep time: 10 minutes | Cook time: 5 minutes | Serves 5

4-pounds (1.8-kg) shrimps, peeled

1 tablespoon dried rosemary

1 tablespoon avocado oil

1 teaspoon apple cider vinegar

1. Mix the shrimps with dried rosemary, avocado oil, and apple cider vinegar.
2. Then sting the shrimps into skewers and put in the air fryer.
3. Cook the shrimps at 400F (205ºC) for 5 minutes.

Per Serving

calories: 437 | fat: 6g | protein: 83g | carbs: 6g | net carbs: 5g | fiber: 1g

Air Fried Mussels

Prep time: 10 minutes | Cook time: 2 minutes | Serves 5

2-pounds (907-g) mussels, cleaned, peeled
1 teaspoon onion powder
1 teaspoon ground cumin
1 tablespoon avocado oil
¼ cup apple cider vinegar

1. Mix mussels with onion powder, ground cumin, avocado oil, and apple cider vinegar.
2. Put the mussels in the air fryer and cook at 395F (202ºC) for 2 minutes.

Per Serving

calories: 166 | fat: 4g | protein: 22g | carbs: 8g | net carbs: 7g | fiber: 1g

Savory Lobster Tail

Prep time: 10 minutes | Cook time: 6 minutes | Serves 4

4 lobster tails, peeled
2 tablespoons lime juice
½ teaspoon dried basil
½ teaspoon coconut oil, melted

1. Mix lobster tails with lime juice, dried basil, and coconut oil.

2. Put the lobster tails in the air fryer and cook at 380F (193ºC) for 6 minutes.

Per Serving

calories: 83 | fat: 1g | protein: 16g | carbs: 1g | net carbs: 1g | fiber: 0g

Delicious Scallops

Prep time: 10 minutes | Cook time: 6 minutes | Serves 4

12 oz scallops
1 tablespoon dried rosemary
½ teaspoon Pink salt
1 tablespoon avocado oil

1. Sprinkle scallops with dried rosemary, Pink salt, and avocado oil.
2. Then put the scallops in the air fryer basket in one layer and cook at 400F (205ºC) 6 minutes.

Per Serving

calories: 82 | fat: 1g | protein: 14g | carbs: 3g | net carbs: 2g | fiber: 1g

Calamari with Hot Sauce

Prep time: 10 minutes | Cook time: 6 minutes | Serves 2

10 oz calamari, trimmed
2 tablespoons keto hot sauce
1 tablespoon avocado oil

1. Slice the calamari and sprinkle with avocado oil.
2. Put the calamari in the air fryer and cook at 400F (205ºC) for 3 minutes per side.
3. Then transfer the calamari in the serving plate and sprinkle with hot sauce.

Per Serving

calories: 36 | fat: 2g | protein: 3g | carbs: 2g | net carbs: 1g | fiber: 1g

Desserts

Chocolate Butter Cake

Prep time: 20 minutes | Cook time: 11 minutes | Serves 4

4 ounces (113 g) butter, melted

4 ounces (113 g) dark chocolate

2 eggs, lightly whisked

2 tablespoons monk fruit

2 tablespoons almond meal

1 teaspoon baking powder

½ teaspoon ground cinnamon

¼ teaspoon ground star anise

1. Begin by preheating your Air Fryer to 370 degrees F (188ºC). Spritz the sides and bottom of a baking pan with nonstick cooking spray.
2. Melt the butter and dark chocolate in a microwave-safe bowl. Mix the eggs and monk fruit until frothy.
3. Pour the butter/chocolate mixture into the egg mixture. Stir in the almond meal, baking powder, cinnamon, and star anise. Mix until everything is well incorporated.
4. Scrape the batter into the prepared pan. Bake in the preheated Air Fryer for 9 to 11 minutes.
5. Let stand for 2 minutes. Invert on a plate while warm and serve. Bon appétit!

Per Serving

calories: 408 | fat: 39g | protein: 8g | carbs: 7g | net carbs: 3g | fiber: 4g

Buttery Chocolate Cake

Prep time: 20 minutes | Cook time: 11 minutes | Serves 4

2½ ounces (71 g) butter, at room temperature

3 ounces (85 g) chocolate, unsweetened

2 eggs, beaten

½ cup Swerve

½ cup almond flour

1 teaspoon rum extract

1 teaspoon vanilla extract

1. Begin by preheating your Air Fryer to 370 degrees F (188ºC). Spritz the sides and bottom of four ramekins with cooking spray.
2. Melt the butter and chocolate in a microwave-safe bowl. Mix the eggs and Swerve until frothy.
3. Pour the butter/chocolate mixture into the egg mixture. Stir in the almond flour, rum extract, and vanilla extract. Mix until everything is well incorporated.
4. Scrape the batter into the prepared ramekins. Bake in the preheated Air Fryer for 9 to 11 minutes.
5. Let stand for 2 to 3 minutes. Invert on a plate while warm and serve. Bon appétit!

Per Serving

calories: 364 | fat: 33g | protein: 8g | carbs: 9g | net carbs: 4g | fiber: 5g

Chocolate Butter Cake

Prep time: 30 minutes | Cook time: 22 minutes | Serves 10

1 cup no-sugar-added peanut butter

1¼ cups monk fruit

3 eggs

1 cup almond flour

1 teaspoon baking powder

¼ teaspoon kosher salt

1 cup unsweetened bakers' chocolate, broken into chunks

1. Start by preheating your Air Fryer to 350 degrees F (180ºC). Now, spritz the sides and bottom of a baking pan with cooking spray.
2. In a mixing dish, thoroughly combine the peanut butter with the monk fruit until creamy. Next, fold in the egg and beat until fluffy.
3. After that, stir in the almond flour, baking powder, salt, and bakers' chocolate. Mix until everything is well combined.
4. Bake in the preheated Air Fryer for 20 to 22 minutes. Transfer to a wire rack to cool before slicing and serving. Bon appétit!

Per Serving

calories: 207 | fat: 17g | protein: 8g | carbs: 6g | net carbs: 3g | fiber: 3g

Butter Chocolate Cake with Pecan

Prep time: 30 minutes | Cook time: 22 minutes | Serves 6

½ cup butter, melted

½ cup Swerve

1 teaspoon vanilla essence

1 egg

½ cup almond flour

½ teaspoon baking powder

¼ cup cocoa powder

½ teaspoon ground cinnamon

¼ teaspoon fine sea salt

1 ounce (28 g) bakers' chocolate, unsweetened

¼ cup pecans, finely chopped

1. Start by preheating your Air Fryer to 350 degrees F (180ºC). Now, lightly grease six silicone molds.
2. In a mixing dish, beat the melted butter with the Swerve until fluffy. Next, stir in the vanilla and egg and beat again.
3. After that, add the almond flour, baking powder, cocoa powder, cinnamon, and salt. Mix until everything is well combined.
4. Fold in the chocolate and pecans; mix to combine. Bake in the preheated Air Fryer for 20 to 22 minutes. Enjoy!

Per Serving

calories: 253 | fat: 25g | protein: 4g | carbs: 6g | net carbs: 3g | fiber: 3g

Baked Cheesecake

Prep time: 40 minutes | Cook time: 35 minutes | Serves 6

½ cup almond flour

1½ tablespoons unsalted butter, melted

2 tablespoons erythritol

1 (8-ounce / 227-g) package cream cheese, softened

¼ cup powdered erythritol

½ teaspoon vanilla paste

1 egg, at room temperature

Topping:

1½ cups sour cream

3 tablespoons powdered erythritol

1 teaspoon vanilla extract

1. Thoroughly combine the almond flour, butter, and 2 tablespoons of erythritol in a mixing bowl. Press the mixture into the bottom of lightly greased custard cups.
2. Then, mix the cream cheese, ¼ cup of powdered erythritol, vanilla, and egg using an electric mixer on low speed. Pour the batter into the pan, covering the crust.
3. Bake in the preheated Air Fryer at 330 degrees F (166ºC) for 35 minutes until edges are puffed and the surface is firm.
4. Mix the sour cream, 3 tablespoons of powdered erythritol, and vanilla for the topping; spread over the crust and allow it to cool to room temperature.
5. Transfer to your refrigerator for 6 to 8 hours. Serve well chilled.

Per Serving

calories: 306 | fat: 27g | protein: 8g | carbs: 9g | net carbs: 7g | fiber: 2g

Crusted Mini Cheesecake

Prep time: 30 minutes | Cook time: 18 minutes | Serves 8

For the Crust:

$1/3$ teaspoon grated nutmeg

1½ tablespoons erythritol

1½ cups almond meal

8 tablespoons melted butter

1 teaspoon ground cinnamon

A pinch of kosher salt, to taste

For the Cheesecake:

2 eggs

½ cups unsweetened chocolate chips

1½ tablespoons sour cream

4 ounces (113 g) soft cheese

½ cup Swerve

½ teaspoon vanilla essence

1. Firstly, line eight cups of mini muffin pan with paper liners.
2. To make the crust, mix the almond meal together with erythritol, cinnamon, nutmeg, and kosher salt.
3. Now, add melted butter and stir well to moisten the crumb mixture.
4. Divide the crust mixture among the muffin cups and press gently to make even layers.
5. In another bowl, whip together the soft cheese, sour cream and Swerve until uniform and smooth. Fold in the eggs and the vanilla essence.
6. Then, divide chocolate chips among the prepared muffin cups. Then, add the cheese mix to each muffin cup.
7. Bake for about 18 minutes at 345 degrees F (174ºC). Bake in batches if needed. To finish, transfer the mini cheesecakes to a cooling rack; store in the fridge.

Per Serving

calories: 314 | fat: 29g | protein: 7g | carbs: 7g | net carbs: 4g | fiber: 3g

Creamy Cheese Cake

Prep time: 1 hour | Cook time: 37 minutes | Serves 8

1½ cups almond flour

3 ounces (85 g) Swerve

½ stick butter, melted

20 ounces (567 g) full-fat cream cheese

½ cup heavy cream

1¼ cups granulated Swerve

3 eggs, at room temperature

1 tablespoon vanilla essence

1 teaspoon grated lemon zest

1. Coat the sides and bottom of a baking pan with a little flour.
2. In a mixing bowl, combine the almond flour and Swerve. Add the melted butter and mix until your mixture looks like bread crumbs.
3. Press the mixture into the bottom of the prepared pan to form an even layer. Bake at 330 degrees F (166ºC) for 7 minutes until golden brown. Allow it to cool completely on a wire rack.

4. Meanwhile, in a mixer fitted with the paddle attachment, prepare the filling by mixing the soft cheese, heavy cream, and granulated Swerve; beat until creamy and fluffy.
5. Crack the eggs into the mixing bowl, one at a time; add the vanilla and lemon zest and continue to mix until fully combined.
6. Pour the prepared topping over the cooled crust and spread evenly.
7. Bake in the preheated Air Fryer at 330 degrees F (166ºC) for 25 to 30 minutes; leave it in the Air Fryer to keep warm for another 30 minutes.
8. Cover your cheesecake with plastic wrap. Place in your refrigerator and allow it to cool at least 6 hours or overnight. Serve well chilled.

Per Serving

calories: 245 | fat: 21g | protein: 8g | carbs: 7g | net carbs: 5g | fiber: 2g

Air Fried Chocolate Brownies

Prep time: 40 minutes | Cook time: 35 minutes | Serves 8

5 ounces (142 g) unsweetened chocolate, chopped into chunks

2 tablespoons instant espresso powder

1 tablespoon cocoa powder, unsweetened

½ cup almond butter

½ cup almond meal

¾ cup Swerve

1 teaspoon pure coffee extract

½ teaspoon lime peel zest

¼ cup coconut flour

2 eggs plus 1 egg yolk

½ teaspoon baking soda

½ teaspoon baking powder

½ teaspoon ground cinnamon

⅓ teaspoon ancho chile powder

For the Chocolate Mascarpone Frosting:

4 ounces (113 g) mascarpone cheese, at room temperature

1½ ounces (43 g) unsweetened chocolate chips

1½ cups Swerve

¼ cup unsalted butter, at room temperature

1 teaspoon vanilla paste

A pinch of fine sea salt

1. First of all, microwave the chocolate and almond butter until completely melted; allow the mixture to cool at room temperature.
2. Then, whisk the eggs, Swerve, cinnamon, espresso powder, coffee extract, ancho chile powder, and lime zest.
3. Next step, add the vanilla/egg mixture to the chocolate/butter mixture. Stir in the almond meal and coconut flour along with baking soda, baking powder and cocoa powder.
4. Finally, press the batter into a lightly buttered cake pan. Air-fry for 35 minutes at 345 degrees F (174ºC).
5. In the meantime, make the frosting. Beat the butter and mascarpone cheese until creamy. Add in the melted chocolate chips and vanilla paste.
6. Gradually, stir in the Swerve and salt; beat until everything's well combined. Lastly, frost the brownies and serve.

Per Serving

calories: 363 | fat: 33g | protein: 7g | carbs: 10g | net carbs: 5g | fiber: 5g

Butter Cake with Cranberries

Prep time: 30 minutes | Cook time: 20 minutes | Serves 8

1 cup almond flour

1/3 teaspoon baking soda

1/3 teaspoon baking powder

¾ cup erythritol

½ teaspoon ground cloves

1/3 teaspoon ground cinnamon

½ teaspoon cardamom

1 stick butter

½ teaspoon vanilla paste

2 eggs plus 1 egg yolk, beaten

½ cup cranberries, fresh or thawed

1 tablespoon browned butter

For Ricotta Frosting:

½ stick butter
½ cup firm Ricotta cheese
1 cup powdered erythritol
¼ teaspoon salt
Zest of ½ lemon

1. Start by preheating your Air Fryer to 355 degrees F (181ºC).
2. In a mixing bowl, combine the flour with baking soda, baking powder, erythritol, ground cloves, cinnamon, and cardamom.
3. In a separate bowl, whisk 1 stick butter with vanilla paste; mix in the eggs until light and fluffy. Add the flour/sugar mixture to the butter/egg mixture. Fold in the cranberries and browned butter.
4. Scrape the mixture into the greased cake pan. Then, bake in the preheated Air Fryer for about 20 minutes.
5. Meanwhile, in a food processor, whip ½ stick of the butter and Ricotta cheese until there are no lumps.
6. Slowly add the powdered erythritol and salt until your mixture has reached a thick consistency. Stir in the lemon zest; mix to combine and chill completely before using.
7. Frost the cake and enjoy!

Per Serving

calories: 286 | fat: 27g | protein: 8g | carbs: 10g | net carbs: 5g | fiber: 5g

Buttery Monk Fruit Cookie

Prep time: 25 minutes | Cook time: 20 minutes | Serves 4

8 ounces (227 g) almond meal
2 tablespoons flaxseed meal
1 ounce (28 g) monk fruit
1 teaspoon baking powder
A pinch of grated nutmeg
A pinch of coarse salt
1 large egg, room temperature.
1 stick butter, room temperature
1 teaspoon vanilla extract

1. Mix the almond meal, flaxseed meal, monk fruit, baking powder, grated nutmeg, and salt in a bowl.
2. In a separate bowl, whisk the egg, butter, and vanilla extract.
3. Stir the egg mixture into dry mixture; mix to combine well or until it forms a nice, soft dough.
4. Roll your dough out and cut out with a cookie cutter of your choice.
5. Bake in the preheated Air Fryer at 350 degrees F (180ºC) for 10 minutes. Decrease the temperature to 330 degrees F (166ºC) and cook for 10 minutes longer. Bon appétit!

Per Serving

calories: 388 | fat: 38g | protein: 8g | carbs: 7g | net carbs: 4g | fiber: 3g

Buttery Cookie with Hazelnut

Prep time: 20 minutes | Cook time: 10 minutes | Serves 6

1 cup almond flour

½ cup coconut flour

1 teaspoon baking soda

1 teaspoon fine sea salt

1 stick butter

1 cup Swerve

2 teaspoons vanilla

2 eggs, at room temperature

1 cup hazelnuts, coarsely chopped

1. Begin by preheating your Air Fryer to 350 degrees F (180ºC).
2. Mix the flour with the baking soda, and sea salt.
3. In the bowl of an electric mixer, beat the butter, Swerve, and vanilla until creamy. Fold in the eggs, one at a time, and mix until well combined.
4. Slowly and gradually, stir in the flour mixture. Finally, fold in the coarsely chopped hazelnuts.
5. Divide the dough into small balls using a large cookie scoop; drop onto the prepared cookie sheets. Bake for 10 minutes or until golden brown, rotating the pan once or twice through the cooking time.
6. Work in batches and cool for a couple of minutes before removing to wire racks. Enjoy!

Per Serving

calories: 328 | fat: 32g | protein: 7g | carbs: 5g | net carbs: 3g | fiber: 2g

Hazelnut Butter Cookie

Prep time: 1 hour | Cook time: 20 minutes | Serves 10

4 tablespoons liquid monk fruit

½ cup hazelnuts, ground

1 stick butter, room temperature

2 cups almond flour

1 cup coconut flour

2 ounces (57 g) granulated Swerve

2 teaspoons ground cinnamon

1. Firstly, cream liquid monk fruit with butter until the mixture becomes fluffy. Sift in both types of flour.
2. Now, stir in the hazelnuts. Now, knead the mixture to form a dough; place in the refrigerator for about 35 minutes.
3. To finish, shape the prepared dough into the bite-sized balls; arrange them on a baking dish; flatten the balls using the back of a spoon.
4. Mix granulated Swerve with ground cinnamon. Press your cookies in the cinnamon mixture until they are completely covered.
5. Bake the cookies for 20 minutes at 310 degrees F (154ºC).
6. Leave them to cool for about 10 minutes before transferring them to a wire rack. Bon appétit!

Per Serving

calories: 246 | fat: 23g | protein: 5g | carbs: 7g | net carbs: 3g | fiber: 4g

Walnut Butter Cookie

Prep time: 40 minutes | Cook time: 15 minutes | Serves 8

½ cup walnuts, ground

½ cup coconut flour

1 cup almond flour

¾ cup Swerve

1 stick butter, room temperature

2 tablespoons rum

½ teaspoon pure vanilla extract

½ teaspoon pure almond extract

1. In a mixing dish, beat the butter with Swerve, vanilla, and almond extract until light and fluffy. Then, throw in the flour and ground walnuts; add in rum.
2. Continue mixing until it forms a soft dough. Cover and place in the refrigerator for 20 minutes. In the meantime, preheat the Air Fryer to 330 degrees F (166ºC).
3. Roll the dough into small cookies and place them on the Air Fryer cake pan; gently press each cookie using a spoon.
4. Bake butter cookies for 15 minutes in the preheated Air Fryer. Bon appétit!

Per Serving

calories: 228 | fat: 22g | protein: 4g | carbs: 4g | net carbs: 2g | fiber: 2g

Buttery Almond Fruit Cookie

Prep time: 50 minutes | Cook time: 13 minutes | Serves 8

½ cup slivered almonds

1 stick butter, room temperature

4 ounces (113 g) monk fruit

$^2/_3$ cup blanched almond flour

$^1/_3$ cup coconut flour

$^1/_3$ teaspoon ground cloves

1 tablespoon ginger powder

¾ teaspoon pure vanilla extract

1. In a mixing dish, beat the monk fruit, butter, vanilla extract, ground cloves, and ginger until light and fluffy. Then, throw in the coconut flour, almond flour, and slivered almonds.
2. Continue mixing until it forms a soft dough. Cover and place in the refrigerator for 35 minutes. Meanwhile, preheat the Air Fryer to 315 degrees F (157ºC).
3. Roll dough into small cookies and place them on the Air Fryer cake pan; gently press each cookie using the back of a spoon.

4. Bake these butter cookies for 13 minutes. Bon appétit!

Per Serving

calories: 199 | fat: 19g | protein: 3g | carbs: 4g | net carbs: 2g | fiber: 2g

Butter and Chocolate Chip Cookie

Prep time: 20 minutes | Cook time: 11 minutes | Serves 8

1 stick butter, at room temperature

1¼ cups Swerve

¼ cup chunky peanut butter

1 teaspoon vanilla paste

1 fine almond flour

⅔ cup coconut flour

⅓ cup cocoa powder, unsweetened

1 ½ teaspoons baking powder

¼ teaspoon ground cinnamon

¼ teaspoon ginger

½ cup chocolate chips, unsweetened

1. In a mixing dish, beat the butter and Swerve until creamy and uniform. Stir in the peanut butter and vanilla.
2. In another mixing dish, thoroughly combine the flour, cocoa powder, baking powder, cinnamon, and ginger.
3. Add the flour mixture to the peanut butter mixture; mix to combine well. Afterwards, fold in the chocolate chips.
4. Drop by large spoonfuls onto a parchment-lined Air Fryer basket. Bake at 365 degrees F (185ºC) for 11 minutes or until golden brown on the top. Bon appétit!

Per Serving

calories: 303 | fat: 28g | protein: 6g | carbs: 10g | net carbs: 5g | fiber: 5g

Blueberry Cream Flan

Prep time: 30 minutes | Cook time: 25 minutes | Serves 6

¾ cup extra-fine almond flour

1 cup fresh blueberries

½ cup coconut cream

¾ cup coconut milk

3 eggs, whisked

½ cup Swerve

½ teaspoon baking soda

½ teaspoon baking powder

⅓ teaspoon ground cinnamon

½ teaspoon ginger

¼ teaspoon grated nutmeg

1. Lightly grease 2 mini pie pans using a nonstick cooking spray. Lay the blueberries on the bottom of the pie pans.
2. In a saucepan that is preheated over a moderate flame, warm the cream along with coconut milk until thoroughly heated.
3. Remove the pan from the heat; mix in the flour along with baking soda and baking powder.
4. In a medium-sized mixing bowl, whip the eggs, Swerve, and spices; whip until the mixture is creamy.
5. Add the creamy milk mixture. Carefully spread this mixture over the fruits.
6. Bake at 320 degrees (160ºC) for about 25 minutes. Serve.

Per Serving

calories: 250 | fat: 22g | protein: 7g | carbs: 9g | net carbs: 6g | fiber: 3g

Air Fried Muffin

Prep time: 5 minutes | Cook time: 25 minutes | Serves 5

½ cup coconut flour

2 tablespoons cocoa powder

3 tablespoons erythritol

1 teaspoon baking powder

2 tablespoons coconut oil

2 eggs, beaten

½ cup coconut shred

1. In the mixing bowl, mix all ingredients.
2. Then pour the mixture in the molds of the muffin and transfer in the air fryer basket.
3. Cook the muffins at 350F (180ºC) for 25 minutes.

Per Serving

calories: 206 | fat: 16g | protein: 4g | carbs: 13g | net carbs: 6g | fiber: 7g

Homemade Muffin

Prep time: 10 minutes | Cook time: 10 minutes | Serves 5

5 tablespoons coconut oil, softened

1 egg, beaten

1 teaspoon vanilla extract

1 tablespoon poppy seeds

1 teaspoon baking powder

2 tablespoons erythritol

1 cup coconut flour

1. In the mixing bowl, mix coconut oil with egg, vanilla extract, poppy seeds, baking powder, erythritol, and coconut flour.
2. When the mixture is homogenous, pour it in the muffin molds and transfer it in the air fryer basket.
3. Cook the muffins for 10 minutes at 365F (185ºC).

Per Serving

calories: 239 | fat: 17g | protein: 5g | carbs: 17g | net carbs: 7g | fiber: 10g

Creamy Pecan Bar

Prep time: 5 minutes | Cook time: 40 minutes | Serves 12

2 cups coconut flour

5 tablespoons erythritol

4 tablespoons coconut oil, softened

½ cup heavy cream

1 egg, beaten

4 pecans, chopped

1. Mix coconut flour, erythritol, coconut oil, heavy cream, and egg.
2. Pour the batter in the air fryer basket and flatten well.
3. Top the mixture with pecans and cook the meal at 350F (180ºC) for 40 minutes.
4. Cut the cooked meal into the bars.

Per Serving

calories: 174 | fat: 12g | protein: 4g | carbs: 14g | net carbs: 5g | fiber: 9g

Lime Bar

Prep time: 10 minutes | Cook time: 35 minutes | Serves 10

3 tablespoons coconut oil, melted

3 tablespoons Splenda

1½ cup coconut flour

3 eggs, beaten

1 teaspoon lime zest, grated

3 tablespoons lime juice

1. Cover the air fryer basket bottom with baking paper.
2. Then in the mixing bowl, mix Splenda with coconut flour, eggs, lime zest, and lime juice.
3. Pour the mixture in the air fryer basket and flatten gently.
4. Cook the meal at 350F (180ºC) for 35 minutes.
5. Then cool the cooked meal little and cut into bars.

Per Serving

calories: 144 | fat: 7g | protein: 4g | carbs: 16g | net carbs: 8g | fiber: 7g

Macadamia Bar

Prep time: 15 minutes | Cook time: 30 minutes | Serves 10

3 tablespoons butter, softened

1 teaspoon baking powder

1 teaspoon apple cider vinegar

1.5 cup coconut flour

3 tablespoons Swerve

1 teaspoon vanilla extract

2 eggs, beaten

2 oz macadamia nuts, chopped

Cooking spray

1. Spray the air fryer basket with cooking spray.
2. Then mix all remaining ingredients in the mixing bowl and stir until you get a homogenous mixture.
3. Pour the mixture in the air fryer basket and cook at 345F (174ºC) for 30 minutes.
4. When the mixture is cooked, cut it into bars and transfer in the serving plates.

Per Serving

calories: 158 | fat: 10g | protein: 4g | carbs: 13g | net carbs: 5g | fiber: 8g

Zucchini Bread

Prep time: 10 minutes | Cook time: 40 minutes | Serves 12

2 cups coconut flour

2 teaspoons baking powder

¾ cup erythritol

½ cup coconut oil, melted

1 teaspoon apple cider vinegar

1 teaspoon vanilla extract

3 eggs, beaten

1 zucchini, grated

1 teaspoon ground cinnamon

1. In the mixing bowl, mix coconut flour with baking powder, erythritol, coconut oil, apple cider vinegar, vanilla extract, eggs, zucchini, and ground cinnamon.
2. Transfer the mixture in the air fryer basket and flatten it in the shape of the bread.
3. Cook the bread at 350F (180ºC) for 40 minutes.

Per Serving

calories: 179 | fat: 12g | protein: 4g | carbs: 15g | net carbs: 7g | fiber: 8g

Creamy Vanilla Scones

Prep time: 20 minutes | Cook time: 10 minutes | Serves 6

4 oz coconut flour

½ teaspoon baking powder

1 teaspoon apple cider vinegar

2 teaspoons mascarpone

¼ cup heavy cream

1 teaspoon vanilla extract

1 tablespoon erythritol

Cooking spray

1. In the mixing bowl, mix coconut flour with baking powder, apple cider vinegar, mascarpone, heavy cream, vanilla extract, and erythritol.
2. Knead the dough and cut into scones.
3. Then put them in the air fryer basket and sprinkle with cooking spray.
4. Cook the vanilla scones at 365F (185ºC) for 10 minutes.

Per Serving

calories: 104 | fat: 4g | protein: 3g | carbs: 14g | net carbs: 6g | fiber: 8g

Homemade Mint Pie

Prep time: 15 minutes | Cook time: 25 minutes | Serves 2

1 tablespoon instant coffee

2 tablespoons almond butter, softened

2 tablespoons erythritol

1 teaspoon dried mint

3 eggs, beaten

1 teaspoon spearmint, dried

4 teaspoons coconut flour

Cooking spray

1. Spray the air fryer basket with cooking spray.
2. Then mix all ingredients in the mixer bowl.
3. When you get a smooth mixture, transfer it in the air fryer basket. Flatten it gently.
4. Cook the pie at 365F (185ºC) for 25 minutes.

Per Serving

calories: 313 | fat: 19g | protein: 16g | carbs: 20g | net carbs: 8g | fiber: 12g

Cheese Keto Balls

Prep time: 15 minutes | Cook time: 4 minutes | Serves 10

2 eggs, beaten

1 teaspoon coconut oil, melted

9 oz coconut flour

5 oz provolone cheese, shredded

2 tablespoons erythritol

1 teaspoon baking powder

¼ teaspoon ground coriander

Cooking spray

1. Mix eggs with coconut oil, coconut flour, Provolone cheese, erythritol, baking powder, and ground cinnamon.
2. Make the balls and put them in the air fryer basket.
3. Sprinkle the balls with cooking spray and cook at 400F (205ºC) for 4 minutes.

Per Serving

calories: 176 | fat: 7g | protein: 8g | carbs: 19g | net carbs: 8g | fiber: 11g

Pecan Butter Cookie

Prep time: 5 minutes | Cook time: 24 minutes | Makes 12 cookies

1 cup chopped pecans

½ cup salted butter, melted

½ cup coconut flour

¾ cup erythritol, divided

1 teaspoon vanilla extract

1. In a food processor, blend together pecans, butter, flour, ½ cup erythritol, and vanilla 1 minute until a dough forms.
2. Form dough into twelve individual cookie balls, about 1 tablespoon each.
3. Cut three pieces of parchment to fit air fryer basket. Place four cookies on each ungreased parchment and place one piece parchment with cookies into air fryer basket. Adjust air fryer temperature to 325°F (163°C) and set the timer for 8 minutes. Repeat cooking with remaining batches.
4. When the timer goes off, allow cookies to cool 5 minutes on a large serving plate until cool enough to handle. While still warm, dust cookies with remaining erythritol. Allow to cool completely, about 15 minutes, before serving.

Per Serving

calories: 151 | fat: 14g | protein: 2g | carbs: 13g | net carbs: 10g | fiber: 3g

Golden Doughnut Holes

Prep time: 10 minutes | Cook time: 6 minutes | Makes 20 doughnut holes

1 cup blanched finely ground almond flour

½ cup low-carb vanilla protein powder

½ cup granular erythritol

¼ cup unsweetened cocoa powder

½ teaspoon baking powder

2 large eggs, whisked

½ teaspoon vanilla extract

1. Mix all ingredients in a large bowl until a soft dough forms. Separate and roll dough into twenty balls, about 2 tablespoons each.
2. Cut a piece of parchment to fit your air fryer basket. Working in batches if needed, place doughnut holes into air fryer basket on ungreased parchment. Adjust the temperature to 380°F (193°C) and set the timer for 6 minutes, flipping doughnut holes halfway through cooking. Doughnut holes will be golden and firm when done. Let cool completely before serving, about 10 minutes.

Per Serving

calories: 103 | fat: 7g | protein: 8g | carbs: 13g | net carbs: 11g | fiber: 2g

Chocolate Chips Soufflés

Prep time: 5 minutes | Cook time: 15 minutes | Serves 2

2 large eggs, whites and yolks separated

1 teaspoon vanilla extract

2 ounces (57 g) low-carb chocolate chips

2 teaspoons coconut oil, melted

1. In a medium bowl, beat egg whites until stiff peaks form, about 2 minutes. Set aside. In a separate medium bowl, whisk egg yolks and vanilla together. Set aside.
2. In a separate medium microwave-safe bowl, place chocolate chips and drizzle with coconut oil. Microwave on high 20 seconds, then stir and continue cooking in 10-second increments until melted, being careful not to overheat chocolate. Let cool 1 minute.
3. Slowly pour melted chocolate into egg yolks and whisk until smooth. Then, slowly begin adding egg white mixture to chocolate mixture, about ¼ cup at a time, folding in gently.
4. Pour mixture into two 4-inch ramekins greased with cooking spray. Place ramekins into air fryer basket. Adjust the temperature to 400°F (205°C) and set the timer for 15 minutes. Soufflés will puff up while cooking and deflate a little once cooled. The center will be set when done. Let cool 10 minutes, then serve warm.

Per Serving

calories: 217 | fat: 18g | protein: 8g | carbs: 19g | net carbs: 11g | fiber: 8g

Creamy Strawberry Pecan Pie

Prep time: 15 minutes | Cook time: 10 minutes | Serves 6

1½ cups whole shelled pecans

1 tablespoon unsalted butter, softened

1 cup heavy whipping cream

12 medium fresh strawberries, hulled

2 tablespoons sour cream

1. Place pecans and butter into a food processor and pulse ten times until a dough forms. Press dough into the bottom of an ungreased 6-inch round nonstick baking dish.
2. Place dish into air fryer basket. Adjust the temperature to 320°F (160ºC) and set the timer for 10 minutes. Crust will be firm and golden when done. Let cool 20 minutes.
3. In a large bowl, whisk cream until fluffy and doubled in size, about 2 minutes.
4. In a separate large bowl, mash strawberries until mostly liquid. Fold strawberries and sour cream into whipped cream.

Spoon mixture into cooled crust, cover, and place into refrigerator for at least 30 minutes to set. Serve chilled.

Per Serving

calories: 340 | fat: 33g | protein: 3g | carbs: 7g | net carbs: 4g | fiber: 3g

Chocolate Chip Cookie Cake

Prep time: 5 minutes | Cook time: 15 minutes | Serves 8

4 tablespoons salted butter, melted

⅓ cup granular brown erythritol

1 large egg

½ teaspoon vanilla extract

1 cup blanched finely ground almond flour

½ teaspoon baking powder

¼ cup low-carb chocolate chips

1. In a large bowl, whisk together butter, erythritol, egg, and vanilla. Add flour and baking powder, and stir until combined.

2. Fold in chocolate chips, then spoon batter into an ungreased 6-inch round nonstick baking dish.
3. Place dish into air fryer basket. Adjust the temperature to 300°F (150ºC) and set the timer for 15 minutes. When edges are browned, cookie cake will be done.
4. Slice and serve warm.

Per Serving

calories: 170 | fat: 16g | protein: 4g | carbs: 15g | net carbs: 11g | fiber: 4g

Homemade Pretzels

Prep time: 10 minutes | Cook time: 10 minutes | Serves 6

1½ cups shredded Mozzarella cheese

1 cup blanched finely ground almond flour

2 tablespoons salted butter, melted, divided

¼ cup granular erythritol, divided

1 teaspoon ground cinnamon

1. Place Mozzarella, flour, 1 tablespoon butter, and 2 tablespoons erythritol in a large microwave-safe bowl. Microwave on high 45 seconds, then stir with a fork until a smooth dough ball forms.
2. Separate dough into six equal sections. Gently roll each section into a 12-inch rope, then fold into a pretzel shape.
3. Place pretzels into ungreased air fryer basket. Adjust the temperature to 370°F (188ºC) and set the timer for 8 minutes, turning pretzels halfway through cooking.
4. In a small bowl, combine remaining butter, remaining erythritol, and cinnamon. Brush ½ mixture on both sides of pretzels.
5. Place pretzels back into air fryer and cook an additional 2 minutes at 370°F (188ºC).
6. Transfer pretzels to a large plate. Brush on both sides with remaining butter mixture, then let cool 5 minutes before serving.

Per Serving

calories: 223 | fat: 19g | protein: 11g | carbs: 13g | net carbs: 11g | fiber: 2g

Pecan Chocolate Brownies

Prep time: 10 minutes | Cook time: 20 minutes | Serves 6

½ cup blanched finely ground almond flour

½ cup powdered erythritol

2 tablespoons unsweetened cocoa powder

½ teaspoon baking powder

¼ cup unsalted butter, softened

1 large egg

¼ cup chopped pecans

¼ cup low-carb, sugar-free chocolate chips

1. In a large bowl, mix almond flour, erythritol, cocoa powder, and baking powder. Stir in butter and egg.
2. Fold in pecans and chocolate chips. Scoop mixture into 6-inch round baking pan. Place pan into the air fryer basket.
3. Adjust the temperature to 300°F (150°C) and set the timer for 20 minutes.
4. When fully cooked a toothpick inserted in center will come out clean. Allow 20 minutes to fully cool and firm up.

Per Serving

calories: 215 | fat: 18g | protein: 4g | carbs: 22g | net carbs: 19g | fiber: 3g

Butter Cheesecake

Prep time: 20 minutes | Cook time: 35 minutes | Serves 6

½ cup blanched finely ground almond flour

1 cup powdered erythritol, divided

2 tablespoons unsweetened cocoa powder

½ teaspoon baking powder

¼ cup unsalted butter, softened

2 large eggs, divided

8 ounces (227 g) full-fat cream cheese, softened

¼ cup heavy whipping cream

1 teaspoon vanilla extract

2 tablespoons no-sugar-added peanut butter

1. In a large bowl, mix almond flour, ½ cup erythritol, cocoa powder, and baking powder. Stir in butter and one egg.
2. Scoop mixture into 6-inch round baking pan. Place pan into the air fryer basket.
3. Adjust the temperature to 300°F (150°C) and set the timer for 20 minutes.
4. When fully cooked a toothpick inserted in center will come out clean. Allow 20 minutes to fully cool and firm up.
5. In a large bowl, beat cream cheese, remaining ½ cup erythritol, heavy cream, vanilla, peanut butter, and remaining egg until fluffy.
6. Pour mixture over cooled brownies. Place pan back into the air fryer basket.
7. Adjust the temperature to 300°F (150°C) and set the timer for 15 minutes.
8. Cheesecake will be slightly browned and mostly firm with a slight jiggle when done. Allow to cool, then refrigerate 2 hours before serving.

Per Serving

calories: 347 | fat: 30g | protein: 8g | carbs: 30g | net carbs: 28g | fiber: 2g

Golden Cheese Cookie

Prep time: 10 minutes | Cook time: 7 minutes | Serves 6

½ cup blanched finely ground almond flour
½ cup powdered erythritol, divided
2 tablespoons butter, softened
1 large egg
½ teaspoon unflavored gelatin
½ teaspoon baking powder
½ teaspoon vanilla extract
½ teaspoon pumpkin pie spice
2 tablespoons pure pumpkin purée
½ teaspoon ground cinnamon, divided
¼ cup low-carb, sugar-free chocolate chips
3 ounces (85 g) full-fat cream cheese, softened

1. In a large bowl, mix almond flour and ¼ cup erythritol. Stir in butter, egg, and gelatin until combined.
2. Stir in baking powder, vanilla, pumpkin pie spice, pumpkin purée, and ¼ teaspoon cinnamon, then fold in chocolate chips.

3. Pour batter into 6-inch round baking pan. Place pan into the air fryer basket.
4. Adjust the temperature to 300°F (150ºC) and set the timer for 7 minutes.
5. When fully cooked, the top will be golden brown and a toothpick inserted in center will come out clean. Let cool at least 20 minutes.
6. To make the frosting: mix cream cheese, remaining ¼ teaspoon cinnamon, and remaining ¼ cup erythritol in a large bowl. Using an electric mixer, beat until it becomes fluffy. Spread onto the cooled cookie. Garnish with additional cinnamon if desired.

Per Serving

calories: 199 | fat: 16g | protein: 5g | carbs: 22g | net carbs: 20g | fiber: 2g

Toasted Coconut Flakes

Prep time: 5 minutes | Cook time: 3 minutes | Serves 4

1 cup unsweetened coconut flakes

2 teaspoons coconut oil

¼ cup granular erythritol

⅛ teaspoon salt

1. Toss coconut flakes and oil in a large bowl until coated. Sprinkle with erythritol and salt.
2. Place coconut flakes into the air fryer basket.
3. Adjust the temperature to 300°F (150ºC) and set the timer for 3 minutes.
4. Toss the flakes when 1 minute remains. Add an extra minute if you would like a more golden coconut flake.
5. Store in an airtight container up to 3 days.

Per Serving

calories: 165 | fat: 15g | protein: 1g | carbs: 20g | net carbs: 17g | fiber: 3g

Cheesy Cream Cake

Prep time: 10 minutes | Cook time: 25 minutes | Serves 6

1 cup blanched finely ground almond flour

¼ cup salted butter, melted

½ cup granular erythritol

1 teaspoon vanilla extract

1 teaspoon baking powder

½ cup full-fat sour cream

1 ounce (28 g) full-fat cream cheese, softened

2 large eggs

1. In a large bowl, mix almond flour, butter, and erythritol.
2. Add in vanilla, baking powder, sour cream, and cream cheese and mix until well combined. Add eggs and mix.
3. Pour batter into a 6-inch round baking pan. Place pan into the air fryer basket.
4. Adjust the temperature to 300°F (150ºC) and set the timer for 25 minutes.
5. When the cake is done, a toothpick inserted in center will come out clean. The center should not feel wet. Allow it to cool completely, or the cake will crumble when moved.

Per Serving

calories: 253 | fat: 22g | protein: 7g | carbs: 25g | net carbs: 23g | fiber: 2g

Cheese Monkey Bread

Prep time: 15 minutes | Cook time: 12 minutes | Serves 6

½ cup blanched finely ground almond flour

½ cup low-carb vanilla protein powder

¾ cup granular erythritol, divided

½ teaspoon baking powder

8 tablespoons salted butter, melted and divided

1 ounce (28 g) full-fat cream cheese, softened

1 large egg

¼ cup heavy whipping cream

½ teaspoon vanilla extract

1. In a large bowl, combine almond flour, protein powder, ½ cup erythritol, baking powder, 5 tablespoons butter, cream cheese, and egg. A soft, sticky dough will form.
2. Place the dough in the freezer for 20 minutes. It will be firm enough to roll into balls. Wet your hands with warm water and roll into twelve balls. Place the balls into a 6-inch round baking dish.
3. In a medium skillet over medium heat, melt remaining butter with remaining erythritol. Lower the heat and continue stirring until mixture turns golden, then add cream and

vanilla. Remove from heat and allow it to thicken for a few minutes while you continue to stir.
4. While the mixture cools, place baking dish into the air fryer basket.
5. Adjust the temperature to 320°F (160ºC) and set the timer for 6 minutes.
6. When the timer beeps, flip the monkey bread over onto a plate and slide it back into the baking pan. Cook an additional 4 minutes until all the tops are brown.
7. Pour the caramel sauce over the monkey bread and cook an additional 2 minutes. Let cool completely before serving.

Per Serving

calories: 322 | fat: 24g | protein: 20g | carbs: 34g | net carbs: 32g | fiber: 2g

Cheesy Cream Puffs

Prep time: 15 minutes | Cook time: 6 minutes | Makes 8 puffs

½ cup blanched finely ground almond flour

½ cup low-carb vanilla protein powder

½ cup granular erythritol

½ teaspoon baking powder

1 large egg

5 tablespoons unsalted butter, melted

2 ounces (57 g) full-fat cream cheese

¼ cup powdered erythritol

¼ teaspoon ground cinnamon

2 tablespoons heavy whipping cream

½ teaspoon vanilla extract

1. Mix almond flour, protein powder, granular erythritol, baking powder, egg, and butter in a large bowl until a soft dough forms.
2. Place the dough in the freezer for 20 minutes. Wet your hands with water and roll the dough into eight balls.
3. Cut a piece of parchment to fit your air fryer basket. Working in batches as necessary, place the dough balls into the air fryer basket on top of parchment.
4. Adjust the temperature to 380°F (193ºC) and set the timer for 6 minutes.
5. Flip cream puffs halfway through the cooking time.
6. When the timer beeps, remove the puffs and allow to cool.

7. In a medium bowl, beat the cream cheese, powdered erythritol, cinnamon, cream, and vanilla until fluffy.
8. Place the mixture into a pastry bag or a storage bag with the end snipped. Cut a small hole in the bottom of each puff and fill with some of the cream mixture.
9. Store in an airtight container up to 2 days in the refrigerator.

Per Serving
calories: 178 | fat: 12g | protein: 15g | carbs: 22g | net carbs: 21g | fiber: 1g

Appendix 1: Measurement Conversion Chart

VOLUME EQUIVALENTS (DRY)

US STANDARD	METRIC (APPROXIMATE)
1/8 teaspoon	0.5 mL
1/4 teaspoon	1 mL
1/2 teaspoon	2 mL
3/4 teaspoon	4 mL
1 teaspoon	5 mL
1 tablespoon	15 mL
1/4 cup	59 mL
1/2 cup	118 mL
3/4 cup	177 mL
1 cup	235 mL
2 cups	475 mL
3 cups	700 mL
4 cups	1 L

VOLUME EQUIVALENTS (LIQUID)

US STANDARD	US STANDARD (OUNCES)	METRIC (APPROXIMATE)
2 tablespoons	1 fl.oz.	30 mL
1/4 cup	2 fl.oz.	60 mL
1/2 cup	4 fl.oz.	120 mL
1 cup	8 fl.oz.	240 mL
1 1/2 cup	12 fl.oz.	355 mL
2 cups or 1 pint	16 fl.oz.	475 mL
4 cups or 1 quart	32 fl.oz.	1 L
1 gallon	128 fl.oz.	4 L

TEMPERATURES EQUIVALENTS

FAHRENHEIT(F)	CELSIUS(C) (APPROXIMATE)
225 °F	107 °C
250 °F	120 °C
275 °F	135 °C
300 °F	150 °C
325 °F	160 °C
350 °F	180 °C
375 °F	190 °C
400 °F	205 °C
425 °F	220 °C
450 °F	235 °C
475 °F	245 °C
500 °F	260 °C

WEIGHT EQUIVALENTS

US STANDARD	METRIC (APPROXIMATE)
1 ounce	28 g
2 ounces	57 g
5 ounces	142 g
10 ounces	284 g
15 ounces	425 g
16 ounces (1 pound)	455 g
1.5 pounds	680 g
2 pounds	907 g

CPSIA information can be obtained
at www.ICGtesting.com
Printed in the USA
BVHW011207150221
600148BV00003B/65